WIT & WISDOM FROM THE YOGA MAT

*125 Peaceful Poses, Mindful Musings
and Simple Tricks for
Leading a Zen Life*

RACHEL SCOTT

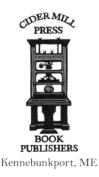

CIDER MILL
PRESS

BOOK
PUBLISHERS
Kennebunkport, ME

13-Digit ISBN: 978-1-60433-675-7
10-Digit ISBN: 1-60433-675-7

This book may be ordered by mail from the publisher. Please include $5.99 for postage and handling.
Please support your local bookseller first!

Books published by Cider Mill Press Book Publishers are available at special discounts for bulk purchases in the United States by corporations, institutions, and other organizations.
For more information, please contact the publisher.

Cider Mill Press Book Publishers
"Where good books are ready for press"
PO Box 454
12 Spring Street
Kennebunkport, Maine 04046

Visit us on the Web!
www.cidermillpress.com

Cover and interior design by Alicia Freile, Tango Media
Typography: Agenda, Amatic, Avenir, Bell, Bodoni Ornament, Cormorant Infant, Eplica, Gotham, and Liorah
All photos used under official license from Shutterstock.com

Printed in China
1 2 3 4 5 6 7 8 9 0
First Edition

CONTENTS

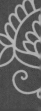

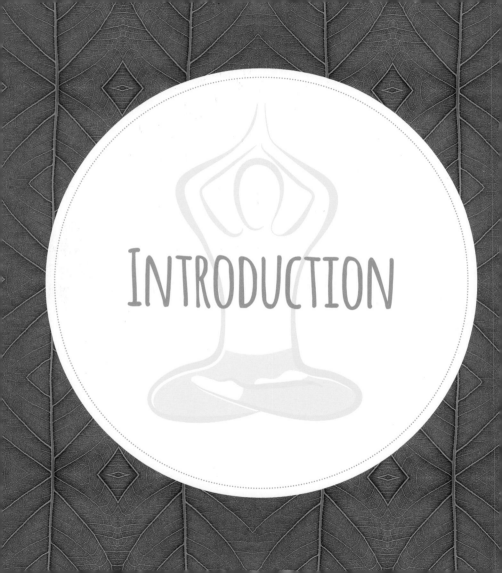

INTRODUCTION

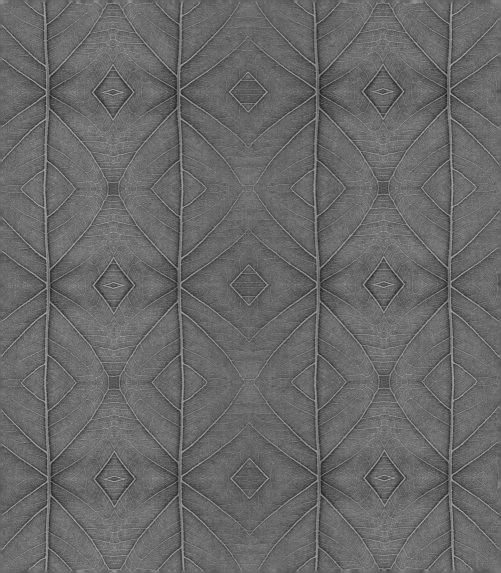

Stress. Our modern epidemic.

I love my technology. Show me a new Apple product and I go a little weak in the knees. But the dizzying rate of information acquisition has also come at a cost. While technological advances have improved our lives in extraordinary ways, we have also become increasingly beset by anxiety, distraction, and materialism. Never far from the Internet, now we are continually "on," "wired," and "plugged in." And while the pace of modern life is exhilarating, it can also leave us feeling weary, burned out, and disconnected.

Yoga couldn't arrive on our shores at a better time.

As our time in cyberspace increases, yoga gives us an essential tether back to the present, living moment. Yoga pulls us out of the virtual world and places us squarely back in our bodies, our breath, and our senses. We are invited to slow down, create some much-needed personal space, and reconnect more deeply to our own hearts. In a world that pulls us continually outwards, yoga reminds us that our most lasting and potent fulfillment resides within.

Yoga is a full-spectrum wellness tool that nourishes our bodies, minds, and spirits. Physically, the asana practice helps us become stronger, more flexible, and more balanced. Mentally, meditation gives us tools to calm our frantic hamster-brain, regain perspective, and let go of stress. Emotionally, we have space to connect to our feelings, share our hearts, and wake up to the vibrancy of our lives.

This book is full of simple and accessible practices that will help you to pause, slow down, and incorporate mindfulness into your daily life. Whether you are new to yoga or a seasoned practitioner, these bite-sized offerings will water the roots of your soul and nourish your deep sense of well-being. Through simple postures, inspirational quotes, and breathing techniques, you will tap into the power of an ancient tradition that has supported practitioners for millennia to recover their poise, vitality, and joy.

I have personally experienced the healing power of yoga. When I took my first yoga class in 1998, I was living in New York City, working as a waitress, and struggling to make my way as an actor. Desperate to prove myself, I managed my anxiety by staying relentlessly busy. I was, to put it mildly, a type-A stress case. A mentor finally took me by the shoulders, looked me straight in the eyes, and said in a very kindly tone, "My dear, please go try yoga. Or perhaps pharmaceuticals. We must calm you down. Please."

At that time, yoga was still a fringe phenomenon, veiled in a hazy smokescreen of incense and intrigue. I crept into my first class nervously, not knowing what to expect. Would I have to contort my body into strange positions? Would they chant things in a weird language? And what the heck was *kundalini* and was it going to rise?

To my surprise, the fundamental teaching of yoga was simple: all I had to do was breathe, move, and feel. Unlike the rest of my life, there was no competition, no judgment, and nothing for me to prove. Yoga provided space to just be. And while that was initially alarming, it proved to be exactly the medicine that I needed. When I stepped out of the studio after class, the city was transformed. I felt the earth beneath my feet

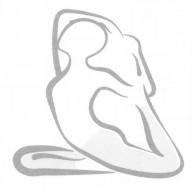

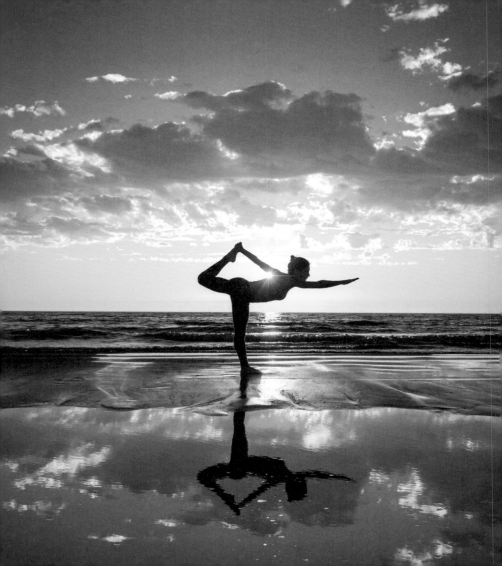

and a new sense of quietude in my heart. My anxiety and restlessness – even for just a short while – had dissolved. I felt like I had come home.

Since that first class, yoga has become a sacred companion, helping me stay centered through all of life's tumults: marriage, death, divorce, job-changes, relationships, loss, and moving to a new country. Yoga has provided the safe and steady space to reconnect to myself and recognize that – even when my world was tilting wildly – I was still okay. Yoga reminds us that we are deeply good, already whole, and perfectly imperfect. As I began to recognize how much yoga was helping me, I became passionate about sharing this wonderful practice with others, and am now a teacher of teachers.

The practices in this book are little gems that help us to come back home to ourselves. Like breadcrumbs, they lead us out of the woods and back to the warmth of our own hearths. When the world around us shifts and storms, yoga reminds us that we are steady, magnificent, and good.

These practices are designed to be incorporated into your busy life when it works for you. Peruse the chapters for a particular meditation or pose that calls to you, or perhaps just open the book randomly and let the Universe decide on your inspiration. While many of these practices can be done in just a few minutes, their effects will remain with you long into your day.

Let the nourishing begin.

See you on the mat,
Rachel

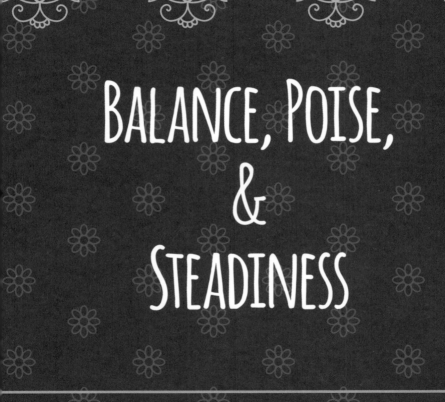

BALANCE, POISE,
&
STEADINESS

We root to rise. What anchors you in your life? Today, nourish your roots to find your greatest expansion.

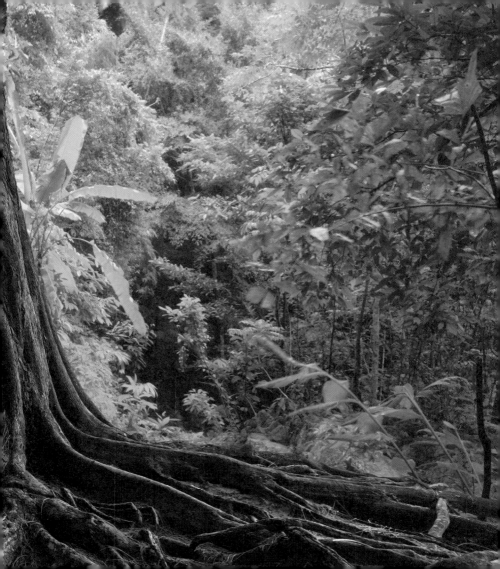

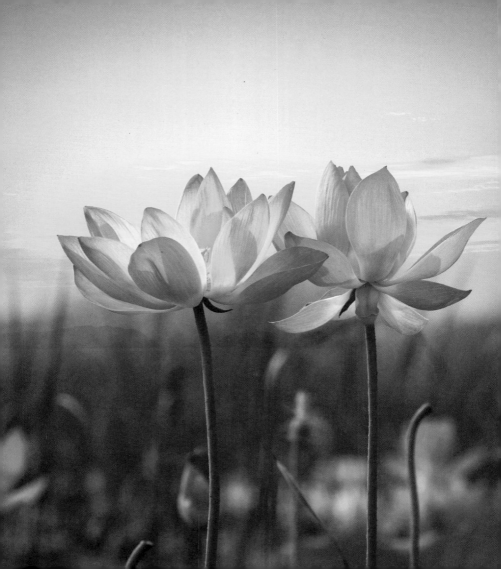

Open to grace.

Delight in discovering your edges.

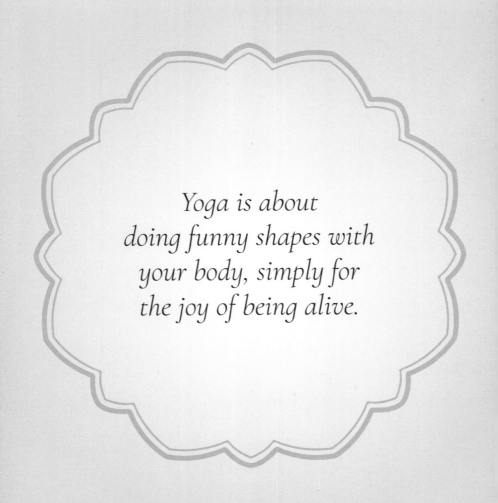

*Yoga is about
doing funny shapes with
your body, simply for
the joy of being alive.*

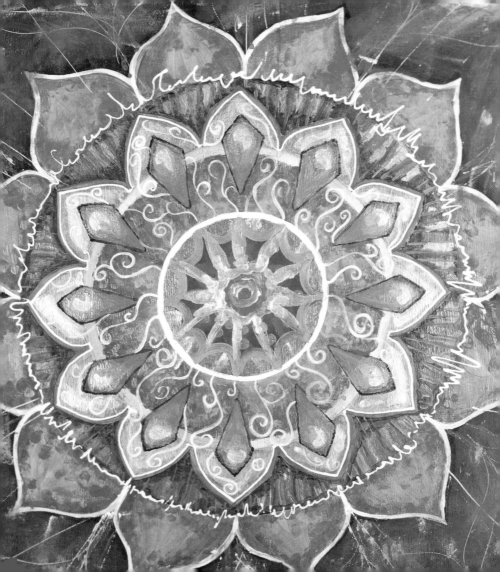

Balance is
never fixed;
it is constant
recalibration.

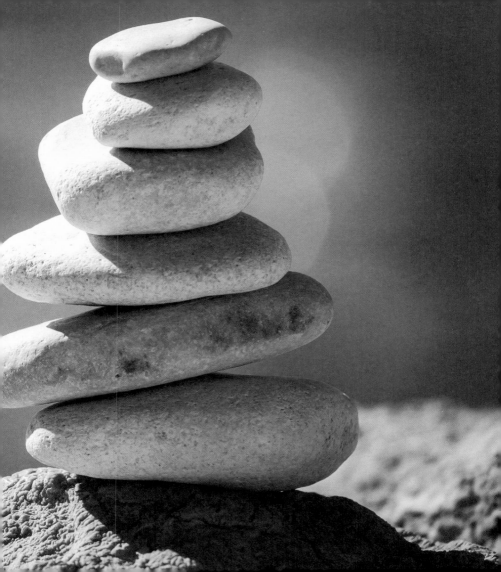

Spanda: the divine vibration of the universe as it continually dances between expansion and contraction. Everything has a fundamental pulse: our heartbeat, the seasons, our feelings, even the planetary orbits.

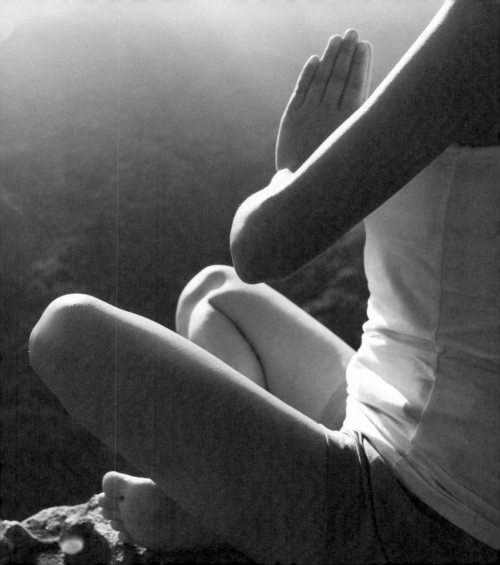

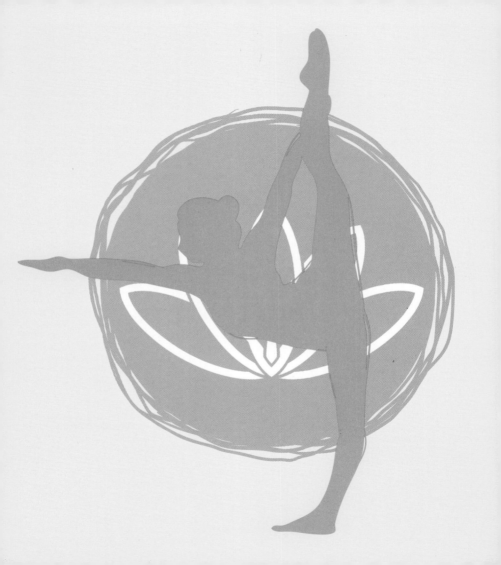

Did you know…

The hatha yoga tradition is rooted in alchemy? Just as alchemists would try to transmute lead into gold, we are participating in a similar process of transmutation when we practice hatha yoga. While we may not literally become gold, we are metaphorically refining ourselves, becoming more lustrous, pure, and radiant from the inside out.

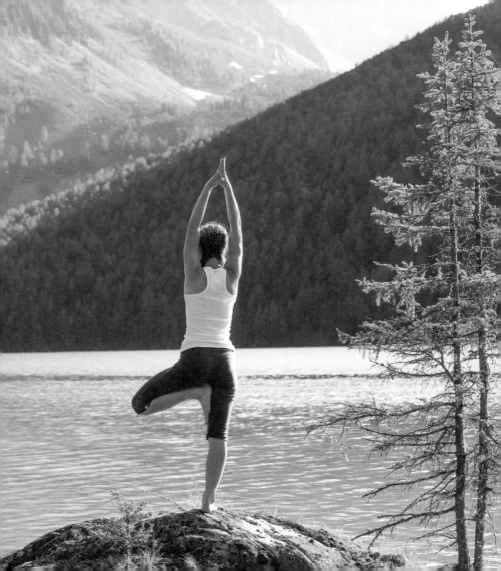

Dare to fall.

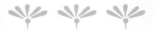

Self-discovery begins
at the edges of
your comfort zone.

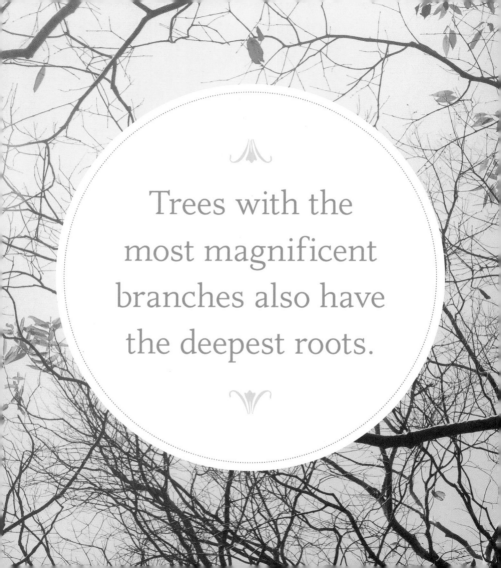

Trees with the
most magnificent
branches also have
the deepest roots.

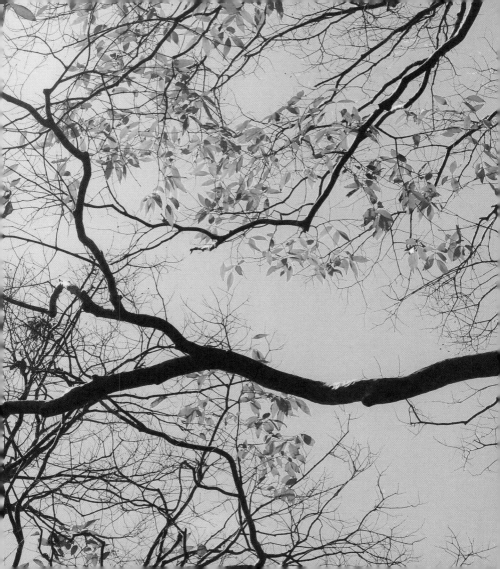

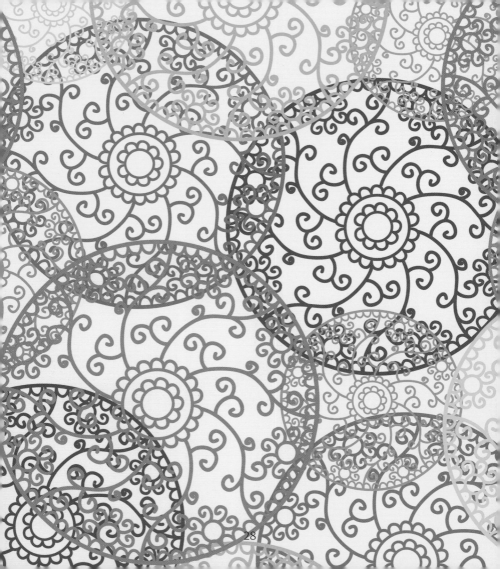

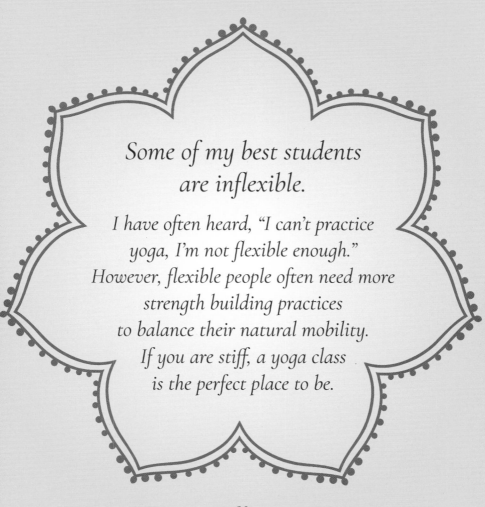

*Some of my best students
are inflexible.*

*I have often heard, "I can't practice
yoga, I'm not flexible enough."
However, flexible people often need more
strength building practices
to balance their natural mobility.
If you are stiff, a yoga class
is the perfect place to be.*

MOUNTAIN POSE

(Tadasana):

FOR CENTERING

Mountain Pose is the foundation for all other yoga poses. Mountain Pose invites us to find our deep roots, connect to our center, and cultivate balanced strength.

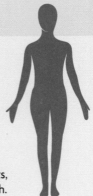

▶ Choose to stand with your feet either hip distance apart or together. Traditional Mountain Pose, practiced with the feet together, cultivates inner strength and connection, while Mountain Pose with the feet hip distance apart cultivates balance and poise.

▶ Ensure your feet are parallel to each other.

▶ Lift all ten toes and feel the inner and outer arches of the feet lift evenly. Keeping the arches lightly engaged, now relax your toes and feel all four corners of your feet anchor to the earth.

▶ Hug your shins towards each other.

▶ Press your feet down as you lift strongly through the muscles of your legs, engaging your quads and hamstrings evenly.

▶ Press the very top of your thighs (where your thigh bone meets your pelvis) back, while you root your tailbone strongly down to the earth. With your hands on your hips, feel that your pelvis is even (so it's not tilting forward, back, or side to side).

- Draw your lower belly slightly in and up to feel the deep support of your core.
- Inhale and lengthen all four sides of your waist.
- Roll your shoulders back and down, and stretch your fingertips down to the earth.
- Soften your front ribs in and down as you draw your shoulder blades slightly together.
- Lengthen through the four sides of the throat so that your chin is level with the floor.
- Soften your eyes.
- Take five to ten deep breaths, feeling the engagement and vibrancy of your body.

HALF MOON

(Ardha Chandrasana):

FOR EXPANSION IN UNCERTAINTY

Feel free to do this at a wall for additional support.

- Start in Warrior II with your right knee bent.
- Bring your right hand to the floor about a foot in front of your right pinkie toe.

- ▶ Bring your left hand onto your hip.
- ▶ Walk your back foot in slightly to shorten your stance and bring most of your weight into your right foot.
- ▶ Come onto the ball of your back foot and straighten your back leg strongly.
- ▶ Look down at your right foot. Press your right knee towards the pinkie toe side of your foot to keep your knee tracking.
- ▶ Keep pressing your right knee wide as you turn your pelvis towards the left side of the mat.
- ▶ Press down strongly through your right foot as you lift your back into the air and level with your hips.
- ▶ Straighten your right leg.
- ▶ Reach strongly through your back heel and lengthen through the crown of your head.
- ▶ If you feel balanced, reach your left hand to the sky and open your chest.
- ▶ If you feel stable, turn to look to the side, or up towards your fingertips.
- ▶ From the center of your body, stretch out into both feet and reach through your arms.
- ▶ Take three to five deep, steady breaths.
- ▶ To come out, look down, bring your left hand to the earth, and lower your left leg to stand in forward fold.
- ▶ Repeat on the second side.

TREE POSE

(Vrksasana):

FOR GRACE IN UNCERTAINTY

Feel free to do this near a wall or use a chair for additional support.

▶ Stand in Mountain Pose (*tadasana*) and place your hands on your hips.

▶ Keeping your hands on your hips, press firmly through all four corners of your left foot and come onto the ball of your right foot. Turn your right knee out about 45 degrees.

▶ Anchoring your left foot into the floor, lift your right foot off the floor and place the sole of your foot on your left ankle, shin, or thigh (above the knee).

▶ Press your foot strongly into your standing leg, and hug your outer hips firmly in.

▶ Lift fully through your torso and through the crown of your head.

▶ Press your palms together in front of your heart (*anjali mudra*).

▶ If you feel steady, root down through your foot and reach your arms overhead to enjoy a full stretch through the length of your body.

▶ For an extra challenge, explore closing your eyes.

▶ To come out, bring your hands back together in front of your heart, turn your right knee forward, and then step your foot down.

▶ Repeat on the second side.

EAGLE

(Garudasana):

FOR STRENGTH IN UNCERTAINTY

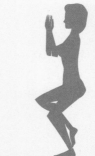

Feel free to do this near a wall or use a chair for additional support.

▶ Stand in Mountain Pose (*tadasana*) and place your hands on your hips.

▶ Bend your knees deeply to come into a Fierce Pose (*utkatasana*, also called "Chair").

▶ Keeping your hands on your hips, press firmly through all four corners of your left foot and come onto the ball of your right foot. Turn your right knee inwards about 45 degrees so that you are knock kneed.

▶ Keeping your deep chair, lift your right leg as high as you can over your left thigh and squeeze the tops of your thighs together.

▶ Hug the right shin either into the left shin, or—joints permitting—wrap the right foot around the left calf.

▶ Squeeze the thighs together as you lengthen your tailbone down and lift your torso to vertical.

▶ Stretch your arms wide, then wrap the right arm under the left. Either hold onto the opposite shoulders, or twine the forearms and press the palms together (option to press the back of the hands together).

- Lift the elbows and press the forearms forward, opening the space between your shoulder blades.

- Root your standing foot into the earth as you wrap the arms and legs together strongly.

- Press into your standing foot, unwind your arms and your legs, and release the pose.

- Repeat on the second side.

WARRIOR III

(Virabhadrasana III):

FOR POWER IN UNCERTAINTY

We will do this version of Warrior III at the wall.

- Stand facing the wall and place your fingertips on the wall at hip height. Make sure your hands are shoulder distance apart.

- As you step your feet back from the wall, press your full palm into the wall and spread your fingers wide.

- Walk your feet back into the room until your ankles are directly under your hips and your body makes an "L-shape."

- Place your feet together and hug your legs together.

- Bend your knees to create space in the backs of your legs.

- Now, as you press your hands firmly into the wall, reach your hips back into the center of the room and stretch your spine fully.
- Lift the back of your neck to keep your head directly between your arms.
- Continue to press your hands vigorously into the wall as you root down through both feet.
- Keeping your right leg straight and strong, lift your left leg up until it's level with your back and you come into a "T" shape.
- Keep your hips square by rolling your inner left thigh to the ceiling and pulling your outer right hip back.
- Stretch fully through the length of your body and breathe.
- Slowly lower the left foot down to come back into an "L-shape."
- Repeat on the second side.

DANCER'S POSE

(Natarajasana):

FOR HEART OPENING IN UNCERTAINTY

Feel free to do this near a wall or use a chair for additional support.

- Stand in Mountain Pose (*tadasana*).

▶ Bend your right knee. Reach back with your right hand, turn your palm open to the right, and hold onto the *inside* of your right foot.

▶ Stretch your left arm to the sky and lengthen through the sides of the waist.

▶ Hug your inner legs towards each other to keep your thighs parallel, then press your right foot back and up into your hand to hinge forward from your hips.

▶ Lengthen your tailbone and engage your core to support your lower back as you reach your heart forward and up and bring your upper back into a backbend.

▶ Square your hips and continue to press your right foot into your hand.

▶ As you anchor into your standing leg, now stretch your body fully out from the center: press your right foot into your hand, reach your left arm up, and use the connection of your back foot into your hand to propel your heart forward and up.

▶ Stay for five to ten deep breaths.

▶ Press firmly into your standing leg and inhale to come up. Release your foot to the earth and feel your body.

▶ Repeat on the second side.

BREATH PRACTICE

FOR CALMING THE NERVOUS SYSTEM

▶ Sit in a comfortable position on a cushion or on a chair.

▶ Place your right hand under your left armpit so that your fingers wrap around your left rib cage.

▶ Cross your left arm over your right, and place your left hand on your right ribs.

▶ Relax your shoulders.

▶ In this position, you will feel the rise and fall of your breath under your hands as you inhale and exhale. When we breathe, we tend to breathe into one side more fully.

▶ Use the feedback from your hands to help you even out the breath so that you are breathing evenly and smoothly into both sides of the ribcage.

▶ If one side of the ribs seems to expand much more than the other, then change the crossing of your arms so that the other arm is on top.

▶ Close your eyes.

▶ Continue to breathe evenly into the left and right sides of the body, bringing balance to your breath.

▶ Slow down your breathing so that the inhale and exhale become smooth and even.

- After about a minute, keep your eyes closed and lower your hands to your thighs.

- Continue to maintain a smooth and balanced breath, feeling the air move generously and evenly into both sides of your lungs.

- Keep a light focus on the balance of your breath into the left and right sides of your body as you allow your breathing to become relaxed and subtle.

- Remain in this light state of focus and balance for several minutes.

- When you are ready, take a few expansive inhalations and exhalations.

- Feel free to stretch or move your body as would feel good.

- Slowly open your eyes.

BREATH PRACTICE

FOR BALANCING RECEIVING AND GIVING

- ▶ Sit in a comfortable position on a cushion or on a chair.
- ▶ Let your hands rest comfortably on your thighs so that your elbows are heavy and your chest is wide.
- ▶ Close your eyes.
- ▶ Inhale and exhale naturally a few times.
- ▶ When you are ready, begin to count your breath. Inhale slowly and mentally count "1-2-3-4."
- ▶ Exhale slowly and mentally count "1-2-3-4."
- ▶ Breathe at a pace that feels natural and calming for you.
- ▶ Keep the inhale and the exhale smooth, calm and even.
- ▶ After a few breaths, you may notice that the rate of your breath naturally becomes slower. If it feels comfortable, slow down your counting and allow your breathing to become deeper.
- ▶ Stay relaxed in your body.
- ▶ Keep a light focus on counting your breath.
- ▶ Remain in this light state of focus and balance for several minutes.
- ▶ When you are ready, take a few expansive inhalations and exhalations.

▶ Feel free to stretch or move your body as would feel good.

▶ Slowly open your eyes.

BREATH PRACTICE

FOR BALANCING THE NERVOUS SYSTEM

Yogis believe that we have a subtle, complex system of energetic pathways (*nadis*) that run through our body. You can think of them like an energetic version of the circulatory system. Two of the most important pathways end in the nostrils—one on each side. The nadi that ends in the left nostril, *ida*, is a conduit for the cooling, feminine, receptive energy of the body, while the nadi that ends in the right nostril, *pingala*, is a conduit for the heating, masculine, active energy of the body. During the day, we naturally alternate which nostril we favor breathing through, indicating the dominance of one kind of energy. By balancing the stimulation of the breath into each nostril during this meditation, we restore our energetic equanimity, balance our nervous system, and calm the mind.

▶ It's a good idea to blow your nose before this practice.

▶ Sit in a comfortable position on a cushion or on a chair.

▶ Bring the index and middle finger of your right hand to lightly touch base the base of your thumb. By doing so, the thumb and ring finger now form a pincer grip. This hands position is called *mrigi mudra*, or "deer seal," because it looks like a deer's antlers and is designed to help us seal and direct energy in our bodies.

▶ Place your thumb on the right side of the bridge of your nose, and your ring finger on the left side. You will find that by applying light pressure to each side, you can control the airflow into each nostril.

▶ Rest your left hand comfortably on your left thigh, with an option to join your thumb and index finger in a circle. This hand position is called *jnana mudra*, or "wisdom seal."

▶ Sit tall, and let your chin soften towards your lifted chest.

▶ Close your eyes.

▶ Inhale and exhale naturally a few times.

▶ When you are ready, close the right nostril and inhale through the left.

▶ Pause, then close the left nostril and exhale through the right.

▶ Inhale through the right.

▶ Pause, then close the right nostril and exhale through the left. This is one complete round.

▶ Inhale through the left.

▶ Exhale through the right.

▶ Inhale through the right.

▶ Exhale through the left. This is two complete rounds.

▶ Continue at your own pace, keeping the breath steady and calm.

- ▶ After about six rounds, finish your last exhale through the left nostril.
- ▶ Rest your right hand on your thigh and join your thumb and index finger in a circle for *jnana mudra*.
- ▶ Take a few natural breaths and sense the deep calm of your body and mind.
- ▶ When you are ready, slowly open your eyes.

Connection, Loving, & Gratitude

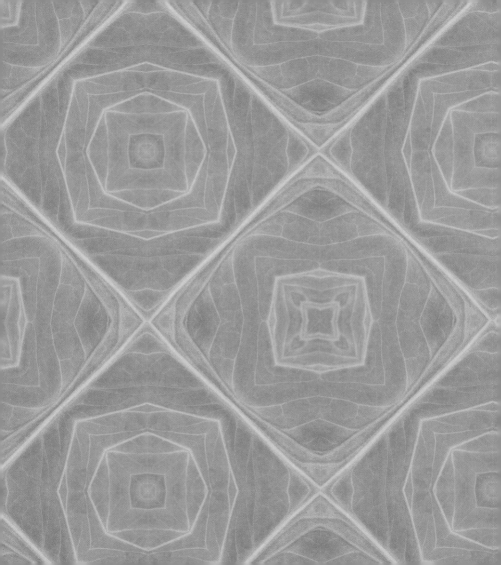

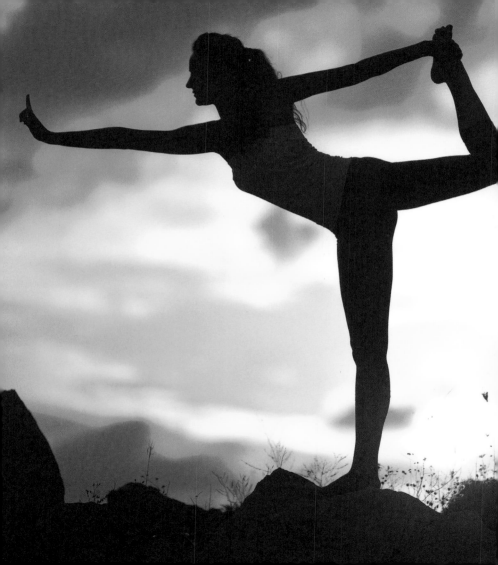

You are not
a problem
to be solved.

You are
already whole.

Today, we are the driver who
is irritated by the oblivious
pedestrian. Tomorrow,
we will be the pedestrian,
irritated by the crazy driver!
When we recognize that
we almost always have been
"the other guy" at one point
or another, we can soften
and remember that we're
all on the same team.

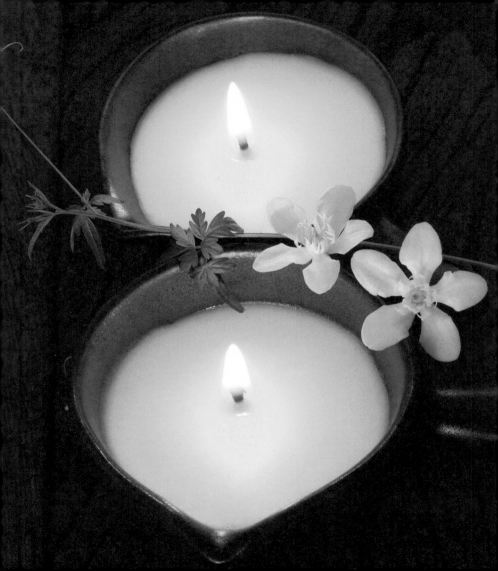

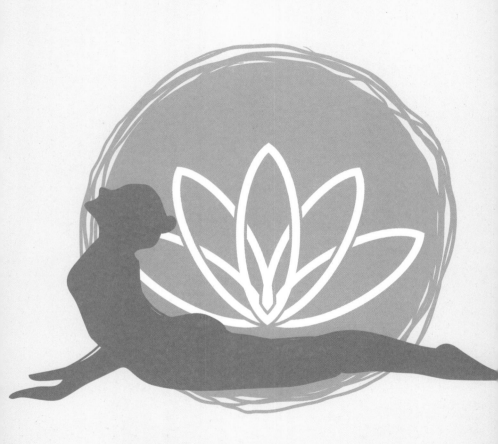

Did you know…

"Hatha" actually means forceful? I like to remind my students of this fact when I hold them in plank pose for a long time.

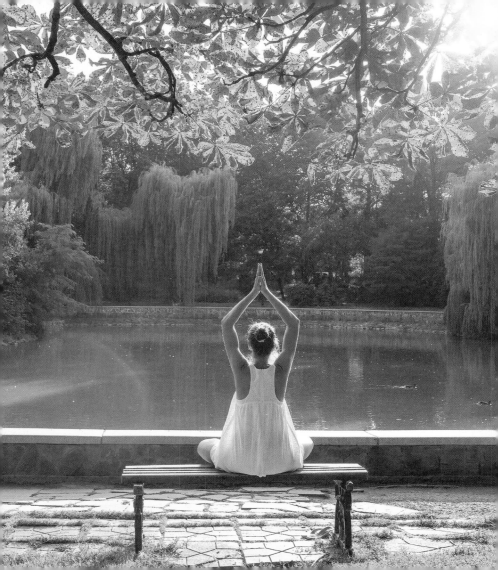

It takes time to share love,
and we often rush
by our opportunities.
Pause for an extra
moment to share your
appreciation for someone.
Spread your love
outwards in little minutes.

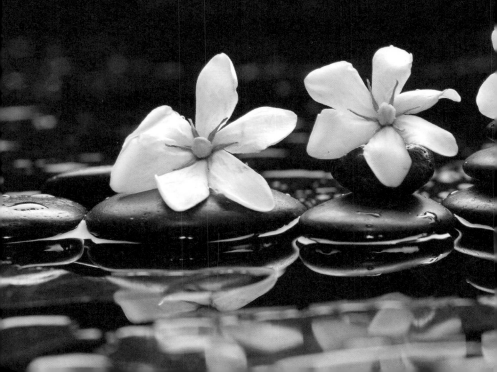

Love is not only
expressed in
grandiose gestures.

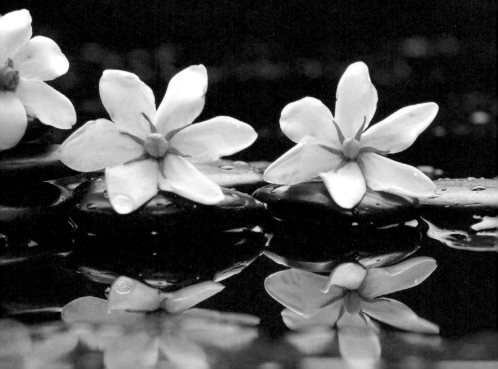

Love is revealed
through our small,
daily acts of kindness.

Love is expressed
through the details.

Through relationships,
we discover ourselves.

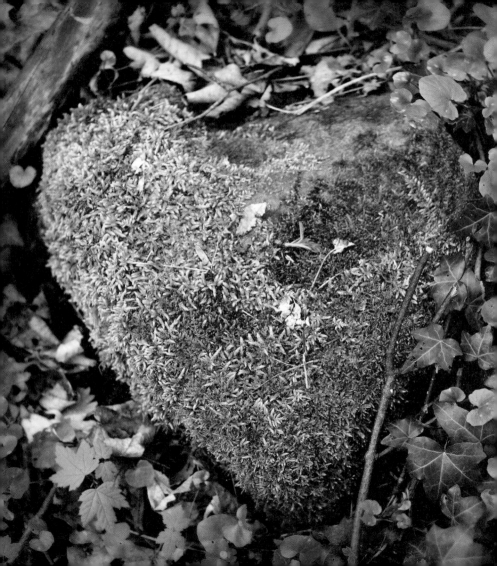

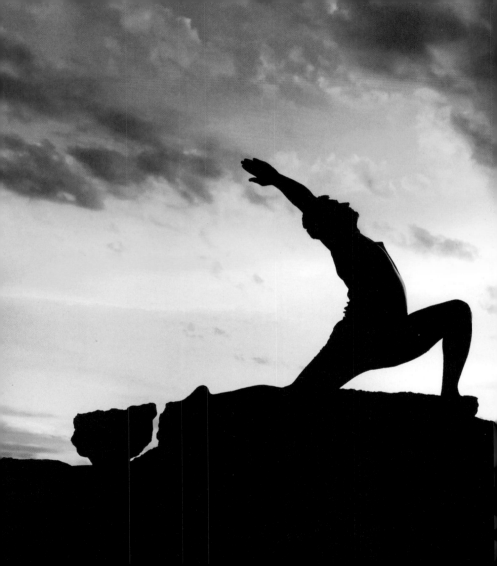

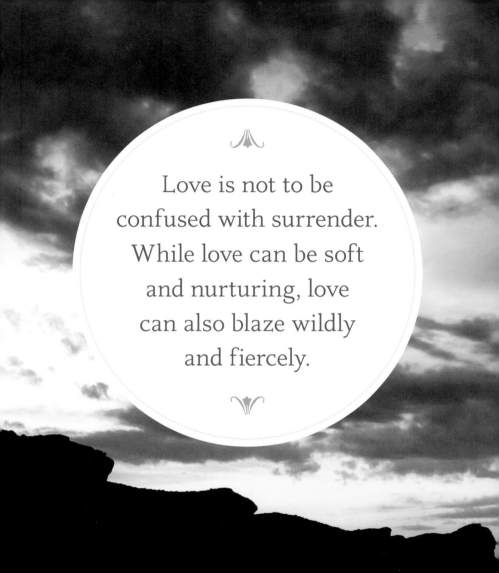

Love is not to be
confused with surrender.
While love can be soft
and nurturing, love
can also blaze wildly
and fiercely.

Is it okay to fall asleep in Savasana?

Yoga confession: I have woken myself up out of Savasana with a ripe old snore. If you fall asleep in Savasana, do not fret. Your body simply needs the rest. Let go. Enjoy.

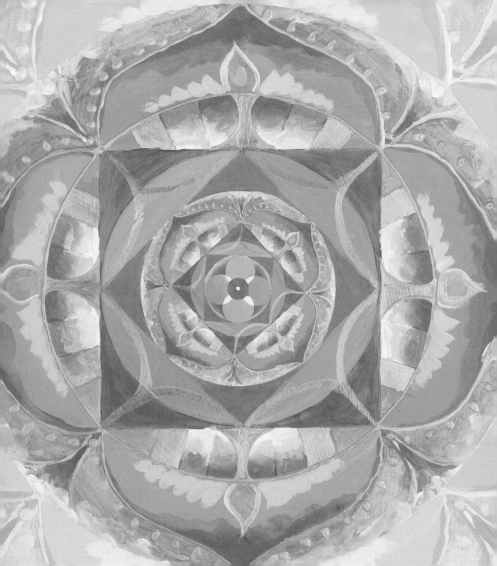

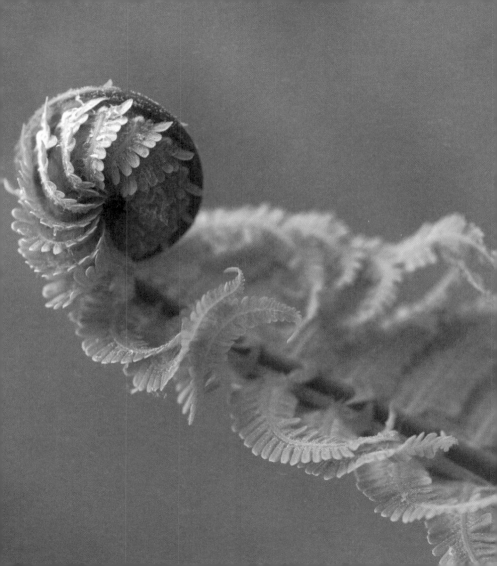

Love is our capacity
to expand, rather than
contract, when faced
with adversity.

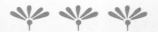

Love means
softening rather
than hardening.

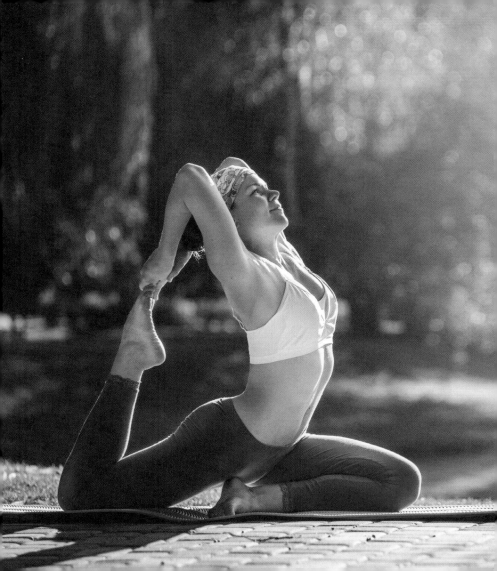

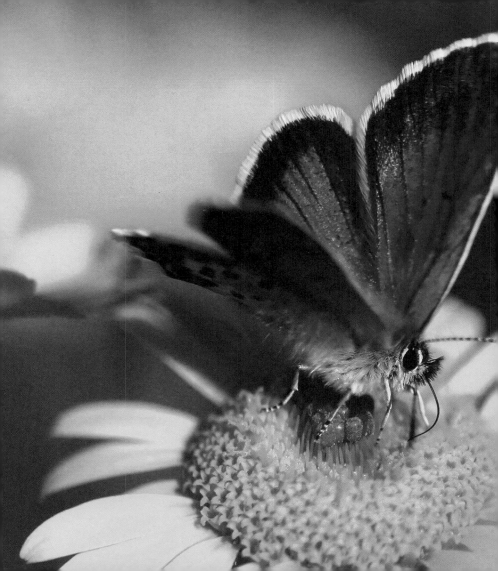

"May all beings everywhere be happy and free."

— MANGALA MANTRA

BRIDGE POSE

(Setu Bandha Sarvangasana):

FOR GROUNDED HEART OPENING

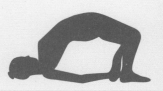

- ▶ Lie on your back, bend your legs, and place your feet flat on the floor so that your ankles are just below your knees.
- ▶ Bend your arms so that your elbows are by your ribs and your fingers are pointing skyward.
- ▶ Press into your heels and inner feet as you lift your hips up.
- ▶ Hug your thighs towards each other to keep the thighs parallel.
- ▶ Lengthen your sitting bones to your knees.
- ▶ Press your upper arms down firmly as you lift your chest towards your chin and open your heart.
- ▶ Press the back of your head lightly down to soften the front of your throat as you gaze to the ceiling.
- ▶ If it feels comfortable, interlace your hands beneath your hips and press your upper arms into the mat to lift your chest.
- ▶ Take three deep breaths.
- ▶ Release your hands and slowly roll down through your spine to lie flat.
- ▶ Take a few breaths.

LUNGE WITH BACKBEND

FOR RADICAL EXPANSION

► From Downward Dog, step one foot forward to your right thumb so that your feet are hip distance apart.

► Place your hand on your front thigh and lift your torso up to come into a high lunge.

► Hug your legs towards each other to create stability.

► Bend your back knee slightly and lengthen your tailbone down to feel your low belly draw in.

► Keep your tailbone lengthened as you begin to lift your back leg to straight.

► Reach your arms forward and up into a wide Y shape.

► As you draw your upper arms back by your ears, lift your heart forward and up to find a backbend in your upper spine.

► Sit more deeply into your front thigh, lift your back leg strongly, and fully stretch through the length of your arms and fingertips.

► Take three deep breaths and feel your inner body expand and open.

► On your final exhale, slowly bring your hands to the floor, step into Downward Dog, and take a few breaths before doing the other side.

SPHINX & COBRA
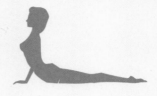

(Bhujangasana):
FOR SOFTENING INTO OPENNESS

▶ Lie on your belly on your mat and prop yourself up on your parallel forearms so that your elbows are under your shoulders (if you feel any discomfort through your low back, then walk your elbows further forward until your lower ribs are connected to the earth).

▶ Press the pinkie toe side of each foot down to feel your upper thighs roll up to the sky so that your legs and feet are parallel.

▶ Press the tops of your feet firmly down and engage your legs strongly.

▶ Lengthen your sitting bones towards your heels to feel the engagement of your core

▶ Pull your bottom ribs in slightly to widen your back.

▶ Exhale to find and retain your core engagement.

▶ As you inhale, roll your shoulders back down and pull your heart forward through the window of your upper arms.

▶ Hug your shoulder blades together and draw your upper arms back to open your chest.

▶ Press your forearms into the earth and energetically pull them towards you, then melt your heart forward.

- **Option:** if your lower back feels supported, then press your hands strongly into the earth and lift your elbows off the floor to move into Cobra pose. Continue to draw your upper arms back and melt your heart forward. Keeping your core engaged and your lower back long, you may explore walking your hands closer in under your shoulders. Stretch through your legs, roll your shoulders back, and soften your heart forward.

- Take three to five deep breaths, feeling your heart widen and soften.

- To come out, slowly lower your upper body to the earth, and then press back into Child's Pose for several breaths.

CAMEL POSE

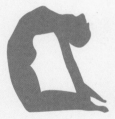

(Ustrasana):

FOR POWERFUL HEART OPENING

- Kneel on your mat with your knees and feet hip distance apart.

- Tuck your toes under and hug your shins towards each other.

- Press the tops of your upper, inner thighs back (it will feel as if you are sticking your bum back slightly and engaging your thigh muscles).

- Keep your quadriceps engaged as you lengthen your tailbone down.

- Lift evenly through all four sides of your torso and bring your hands to your hips.

- Draw your lower belly in and up to your lower back as you draw your shoulders back and down.

- Keeping your body in one long line from your knees to the crown of your head (no backbend yet), hinge the length of your body back from your knees and then rise back up. You will feel your core and your legs working strongly to support you.

- On your third time leaning back, reach back and grasp your heels with your hands.

- Keeping your chin tucked to your chest, start to lift your heart up to the sky and move the backbend into your upper back.

- Lengthen your tailbone to the earth and hug the fronts of your thighs together strongly so that they stay parallel.

- Tuning in to the sensation in your back, begin to press the pelvis forward to bring a long, luxurious, and even curve through your spine. As every spine is different, honor the position that feels expansive through your heart and supported in your lower back.

- Breathe.

- To come out, shift your hips slightly back towards your ankles to come out of the backbend, engage your core, and lift the length of your body up in one piece.

- Sit on your heels, close your eyes, and enjoy the aftereffects of this strong pose.

MEDITATION

FOR LOVING YOURSELF

- ▶ Take a comfortable seat on the floor or a chair.

- ▶ Place your left hand over your heart center and your right hand over your left and feel your heartbeat.

- ▶ Take a few easy breaths.

- ▶ Feel the warmth of your hands moving into your heart.

- ▶ Visualize a soft white light at the center of your chest beneath your hands.

- ▶ As you inhale, visualize this radiant light expanding outward from your heart and nourishing everything nearby in kindness and health.

- ▶ As you exhale, visualize this light softening back to your heart center.

- ▶ With every inhale, allow the radius of the light to grow until eventually every cell in your body is suffused and nourished with its love and well-being.

- ▶ After a few minutes, release the visualization and simply rest in the afterglow of your practice for several breaths.

- ▶ Bow your head to your heart in gratitude for your body's well-being and infinite intelligence.

MEDITATION

FOR LOVING OTHERS

▶ Take a comfortable seat on the floor or a chair.

▶ Place your hands on your thighs and draw your upper arms back to widen your heart.

▶ Take a few easy breaths.

▶ Bring to mind a person for whom you find it easy to feel love.

▶ As you picture this person, think to yourself, "Just like me, you want to be happy." Repeat this phrase silently to yourself several times, and feel your love for this person radiate through your body.

▶ Next, bring to mind someone about whom you feel neutral.

▶ As you picture this person, think to yourself "Just like me, you want to be happy." Repeat this phrase silently to yourself several times, feeling your compassion for this person expand and grow.

▶ Finally, bring to mind someone whom you can experience as challenging.

▶ Again, think, "Just like me, you want to be happy." Repeat this phrase several times silently to yourself, and sense a softening and greater compassion for this individual and their struggles.

- ▶ Expand your meditation out to the world, encompassing all beings, "Just like me, you want to be happy."

- ▶ Stay in this meditation for several minutes, feeling the kindness of your heart flow out to the world.

- ▶ Take a few slow breaths.

- ▶ Sense the well-being and kindness that you have fostered flow through your body.

- ▶ Bring your palms together at your sternum, and bow your head to your gracious heart.

MEDITATION

FOR LOVING YOUR BODY

During the meditation, we take the time to acknowledge our beautiful bodies and our aliveness. For each part of the body that you visit, you can create your own personalized statement of gratitude; the following are merely suggestions for where to start. You also may wish to place your hands on your body as you travel through your gratitude map. During the meditation, feel free to venture all around your body, expressing your gratitude for as many places as you can imagine.

▶ Take a comfortable seat on the floor or a chair.

▶ Place your hands on your thighs either palms up (to feel more opening) or palms down (to feel more grounding).

▶ Close your eyes.

▶ Take a few easy breaths.

▶ Place your hands on your heart.

▶ Starting with your heart, repeat to yourself, "Thank you heart, for all the work you do to keep me alive. Your power, your steadiness. What a miracle to have such a wonderful heart. Thank you!"

▶ Remain with your heart for a few breaths, sending love to your body.

▶ Place your hands on head.

- "Thank you, beautiful brain, for all the work you do to keep me alive. Thank you for helping me think, remember, imagine, speak. What a miracle to have such a wonderful brain. Thank you!"

- Place your hands over your eyes.

- "Thank you, beautiful eyes, for helping to me see the world and everything that I love in it. What a miracle to have such wonderful eyes. Thank you!"

- Place your hands over your ears.

- "Thank you, beautiful ears, for helping me hear the world and everything that I love in it. What a miracle to have such wonderful ears. Thank you!"

- Continue your progression of gratitude through your body, thanking any part that you wish. It's wonderful to thank your bones, organs, muscles, blood, and cells for everything that they do.

- When you have completed your gratitude journey, come back and bring your hands to your heart.

- "Thank you, my whole body, for your miraculous work to keep me alive. To allow me to be, move, and feel in the world. What a miracle to have such a wonderful body. Thank you."

- Pause and take a few deep breaths, saturated in the knowledge that you truly are a miracle of creation.

Empowering
&
Transformational

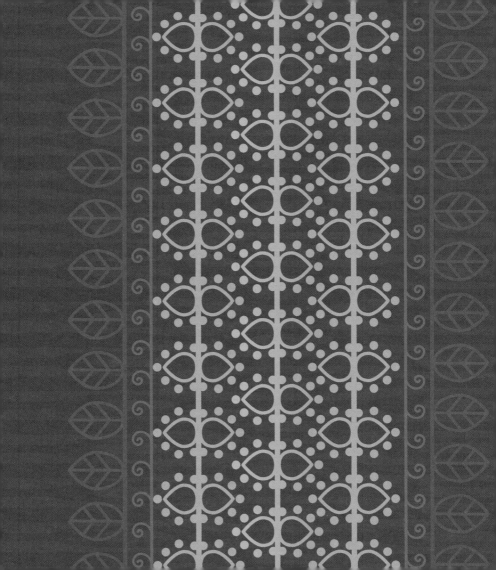

Tapas: a Sanskrit word that describes the heat and friction necessary for change. Tapas is our willingness to endure intensity for the sake of transformation.

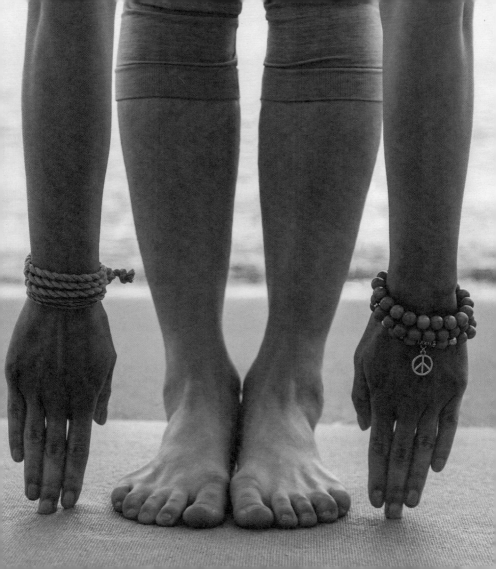

Clear your space to clear your mind.

❋ ❋ ❋

Showing up
is the most
important step.

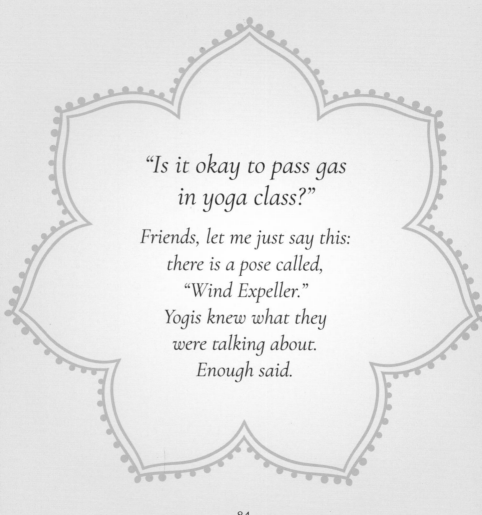

"Is it okay to pass gas
in yoga class?"

Friends, let me just say this:
there is a pose called,
"Wind Expeller."
Yogis knew what they
were talking about.
Enough said.

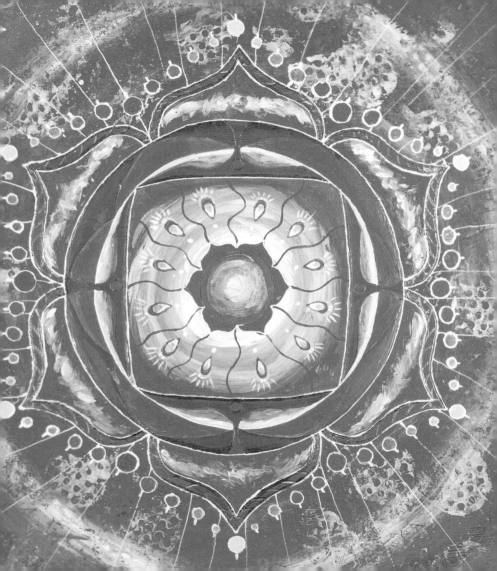

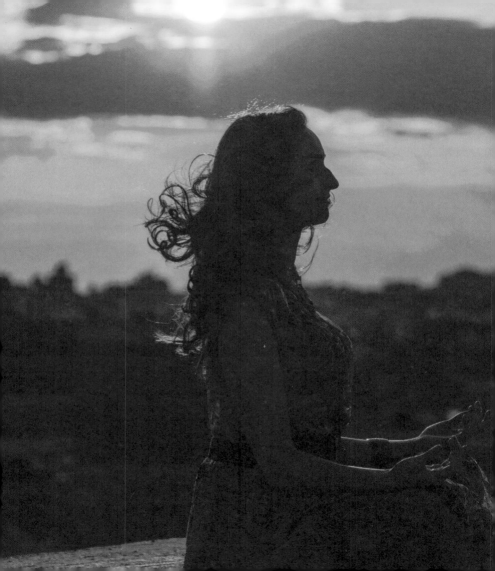

You are stronger
than you know.

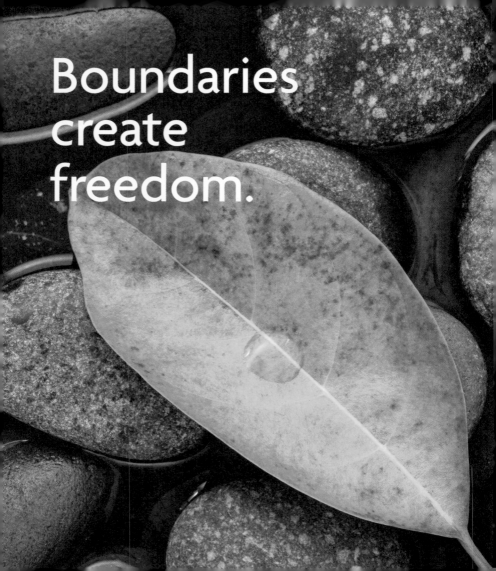

Boundaries
create
freedom.

To many of us, boundaries seem harsh, as if they were an imposed separation or division. This is a confusion. Boundaries are loving and flexible membranes that are necessary for health and vitality. Think of our cells, discerning what will bring health and ease, and what will bring discord. In the same way, our capacity to hold mindful boundaries allows us to uphold a nourishing environment for both ourselves and for others.

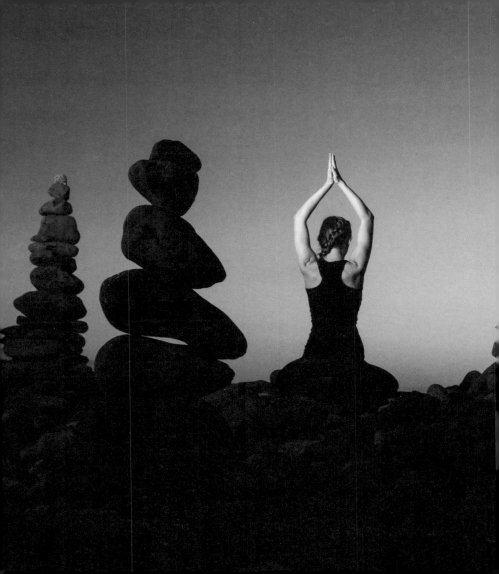

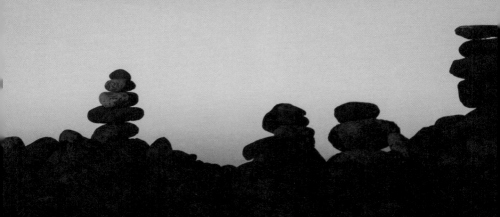

"Do, or do not.
There is no try."

– YODA

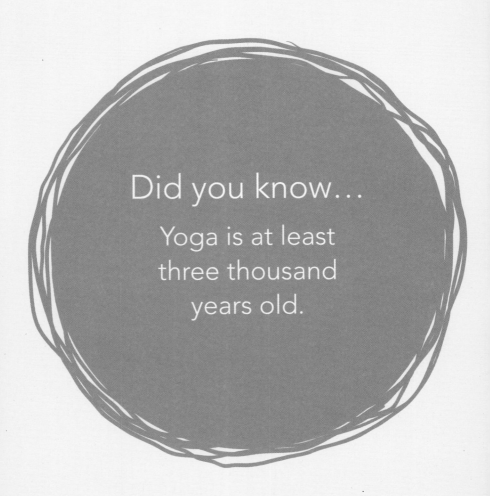

Did you know…

Yoga is at least
three thousand
years old.

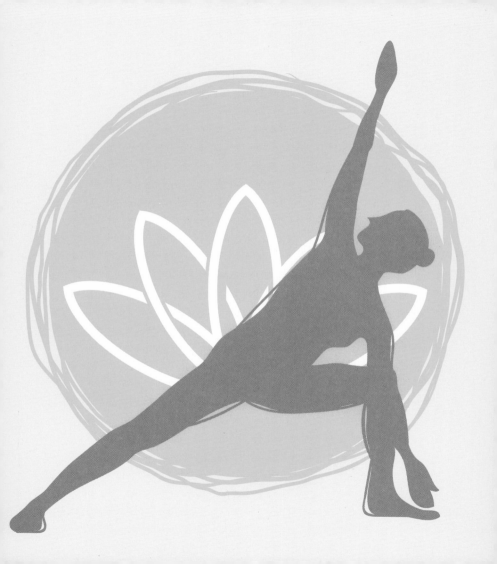

Let go of self-limiting beliefs.

Don't believe everything you think.

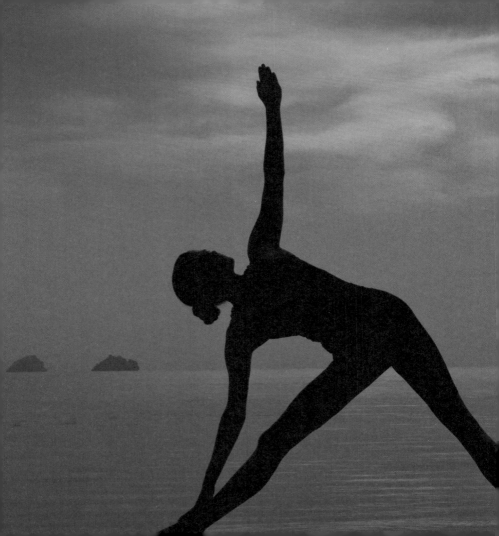

Lean into uncertainty.

DOWNWARD FACING DOG

(Adho Mukha Svanasana):

THE EVERYTHING POSE

Downward Dog opens the spine, shoulders, hamstrings, and calves. It is both a forward fold and an inversion, inviting us to turn the world upside down and change our perspective. While Downward Dog initially requires a great deal of fortitude and flexibility, with practice it also becomes increasingly calming and centering.

▶ Start from your hands and knees, with your hands outer-shoulder distance apart and your feet just behind your knees.

▶ Turn your hands out slightly so that your index finger is pointed straight forward, and spread your fingers wide.

▶ Press strongly through the tips of your fingers and base of your knuckles to take weight off of your wrists.

▶ Curl your toes under and lift your knees up a few inches.

▶ Keeping your knees bent, stretch your hips up and back until are fully extended in one line from your fingertips through your hips.

▶ Press your index knuckles down and hug your forearms towards each other to fully straighten your arms.

▶ Roll your upper, inner arms up to the sky so that the muscles across the back of your neck become soft and spacious.

- Keeping your spine long, lift the muscles of your thighs up strongly.

- As you lift strongly through the fronts of your thighs, sink the center of your heels towards the floor so that your legs move towards becoming straight.

- Ensure that your feet are parallel, so that the center of your heel disappears behind the ball of your foot.

- Press through your hands, stretch your hips up and back, and reach your heels down to fully lengthen and expand your body.

- Take five to ten deep breaths, feeling your inner body open and stretch.

- On your next exhale, slowly lower your knees to the earth and set your hips back on your heels to come into Child's Pose.

WARRIOR II

(Virabhadrasana II):

FOR FINDING YOUR CENTERED STRENGTH

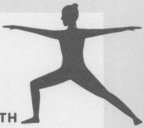

- Stand in the center of your mat and turn so that you are facing the long side.

- Lift your arms wide to shoulder height, stretch through your fingertips, and hug the muscles of your arms to the bone.

- Step your feet wide apart, so that your ankles are under your wrists.

- From the top of your right thigh, turn your right leg out ninety degrees so that your right toes point to the short end of the mat.

- Align the center of your right heel with the arch of your left foot.

- Turn your left toes in slightly.

- Anchor strongly through your left heel as you bend your right knee to a square, bringing your right knee directly over your right ankle.

- Lift the front of your pelvis up so that the "bowl" of the pelvis is even and not spilling.

- Press your left outer foot firmly as you wrap your right sitting bone down to the floor.

- Engage your core, widen your back ribs, and lengthen through the sides of your waist.

- Pull your heels towards each other to engage your legs as you sit more deeply into the pose.

- Draw your shoulder blades down your back, stretch your arms wide at shoulder height, and turn your head to gaze softly over your right fingertips.

- Take five slow, steady breaths to relish the strength and power of your body.

- Slowly straighten your right leg and turn the right thigh forward to parallel.

- Lower your hands to your hips.

- Take a smooth breath.

- Repeat on the left side.

FIERCE POSE

(Utkatasana):

FOR FINDING YOUR POWER (ALSO KNOWN AS "CHAIR")

- ▶ Bring your toes together and your heels slightly apart so that your feet are parallel.

- ▶ Hug your shins and thighs together strongly.

- ▶ Bend your knees, hinge forward from your hips, and send your bum back and down to sit into Fierce Pose.

- ▶ Lift your toes momentarily to ensure your weight is firmly anchored into the center of your heels.

- ▶ Lengthen your sitting bones down until you feel a lift through the lower belly.

- ▶ Draw your lower ribs in to keep your back body wide.

- ▶ Reach your arms forward and up.

- ▶ Soften your shoulders away from your ears as you strongly straighten your arms and hug your outer arms towards each other.

- ▶ Breathe and sit deeper into the pose to strengthen your legs, back, and shoulders.

- ▶ Remain for five slow breaths.

▶ Stand and release your arms to your sides to come out.

▶ Take a breath and enjoy the strength of your body.

SIDE ANGLE POSE

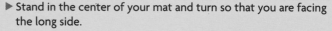

(Parsvakonasana):

FOR CULTIVATING FORTITUDE

OPTIONAL PROPS: block

▶ Stand in the center of your mat and turn so that you are facing the long side.

▶ Lift your arms wide to shoulder height.

▶ Step your feet wide apart, so that your ankles are under your wrists.

▶ From the top of your right thigh, turn your right leg out ninety degrees so that your right toes point to the short end of the mat.

▶ Align the center of your right heel with the arch of your left foot.

▶ Turn your left toes in slightly.

▶ Anchor strongly through your left heel as you bend your right knee to a square, bringing your right knee directly over your right ankle.

▶ Shift your hips towards your back heel and place your right forearm on your right thigh.

- Look down and ensure that your right knee is still over your ankle. If you have a block, you may place your right hand on a block to the outside of your front foot.
- Press your knee towards the pinkie toe side of your front foot and feel your right hip pull back and wrap under you.
- Lengthen your sitting bones towards your back heel and draw your front ribs in.
- Press your right forearm down and draw your right shoulder blade onto your back as you stretch your left arm up to the sky and turn your chest slightly towards the sky.
- Turn your left palm towards the front of your mat. Keeping your left shoulder anchored onto your back, sweep your left arm over your ear.
- Press strongly through your back heel and stretch through your top arm to lengthen your whole body.
- Take five slow and strong breaths and enjoy your strength.
- After your last exhale, press into your front heel and inhale to lift your torso up.
- Straighten your right leg.
- Turn the right thigh forward to parallel.
- Lower your hands to your hips.
- Take a smooth breath.
- Repeat on the left side.

LOCUST POSE

(Salabhasana):

FOR FULL BODY STRENGTH

OPTIONAL PROPS: strap

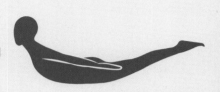

- ▶ Lie on your belly on your mat with your forehead on the floor and your hands by your sides.

- ▶ Lift one leg at a time and stretch it back behind you.

- ▶ Press the pinkie toe side of each foot down to feel your upper thighs roll up to the sky so that your legs are parallel.

- ▶ Press the tops of your feet firmly down and lift your quadriceps strongly.

- ▶ Lengthen your sitting bones towards your heels to feel the engagement of your core.

- ▶ Interlace your hands behind your back (or hold onto a strap with your palms facing down).

- ▶ Roll your shoulders down your back.

- ▶ Exhale to find and retain your engagement.

- ▶ As you inhale lift your chest.

- ▶ Stretch your hands towards your heels to lift your chest as you pull your heart forward.

- Look down and lengthen the back of your neck to lift your heart higher.
- If you are feeling supported through your lower back, reach back through your toes and lift your legs up.
- Firmly engage your thighs and hug them towards each other to keep your legs parallel.
- Inhale and stretch and lift the whole length of your body.
- Stay for three breaths, breathing strongly into your upper chest.
- On your final exhale, lower your body, release your hands, turn your head to one side, and completely let go.
- Repeat the pose once more, changing the interlace of your hands.
- When you have finished, take a few breaths in Child's Pose.

TWISTED LUNGE

(Parivrtta Parsvakonasana):
POSE FOR TRANSFORMATION

- Stand with your feet hip distance apart and parallel.
- Soften your knees and forward fold, bringing your hands to the earth.
- Lower your back knee lightly down and tuck your back toes under.

- ▶ Bring your palms together in front of your chest, and press them together to widen your heart.

- ▶ Inhale and lengthen your spine.

- ▶ Squeeze your legs together for stability and bring your left elbow to the outside of your right knee.

- ▶ Press your elbow into your knee to turn your belly and chest to the right.

- ▶ Hug your right hip back and lengthen the top waist to make your torso even.

- ▶ Draw your shoulder blades onto your back and pull your hands towards the left side of your chest.

- ▶ If you feel stable, hug your legs and lift your back thigh strongly off the floor.

- ▶ Inhale to lengthen, and exhale to twist.

- ▶ Take three deep breaths to feel the power through your legs and your core.

- ▶ Inhale to untwist and bring your hands to the earth.

- ▶ Step forward into forward fold and take a breath.

- ▶ When you are ready, step your right foot back and repeat on the left side.

FOREARM PLANK/PLANK

Set a timer for this pose (30 seconds, 1 minute, 2 minutes) and watch your strength increase over time. This pose can also be practiced on the forearms (forearm plank) or the hands (plank).

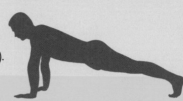

▶ Come onto your hands and knees.

▶ Place your elbows underneath your shoulders and interlace your fingers.

▶ Press your forearms firmly into your mat and step one foot back at a time to come into forearm plank.

▶ Lift your hips to the level of your shoulders, and then lengthen your tailbone back to your heels to engage your core and support your lower back.

▶ Engage the muscles of your thighs strongly.

▶ Press your forearms down.

▶ Lift your front ribs in as you draw your shoulder blades closer together on your back and widen your chest.

▶ Press back through your heels as you reach your heart forward.

▶ When your time is complete, lower your knees softly to your mat, press back into Child's Pose, and take a few deep breaths.

UPWARD FACING DOG

(Urdhva Mukha Svanasana):

FOR EMPOWERED HEART OPENING

A traditional pose of the sun salutations,
Upward Facing Dog uses the strength
of your legs, core, and arms to create
a strong platform for opening the heart.
Practice Upward Facing Dog after mastering
Cobra and Sphinx.

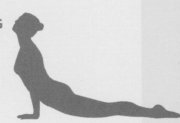

▶ Start on your belly and bring your hands under shoulders.

▶ Lift one leg at a time and reach it back behind you.

▶ Press the pinkie toe side of each foot down to feel your upper thighs roll up to the sky so that your legs are parallel.

▶ Press the tops of your feet firmly down and engage your legs strongly.

▶ Lengthen your sitting bones towards your heels to feel the engagement of your core.

▶ Lift your shoulders to the sky and roll them down your back.

▶ Engage your core strongly.

▶ Press into your hands and lift your chest to come into baby Cobra.

- ▶ Press strongly through your hands and straighten your arms fully as you lift your legs and pelvis off of the floor.
- ▶ Root strongly through the tops of your feet to engage your legs.
- ▶ Soften your elbows slightly to pull your upper arm bones back strongly, and reach your heart forward and up.
- ▶ Lengthen the back of your neck and gaze to your nose.
- ▶ Take three breaths into your upper chest.
- ▶ To come up, draw your core in and up and lift your pelvis up and back to Downward Dog.
- ▶ Lower your knees and come into Child's Pose.

BREATH PRACTICE

(Kapalabhati):

BREATH FOR FINDING YOUR INNER FIRE

Also called "skull shining," *kapalabhati* is a breathing practice designed to tone the core, invigorate the body, and enliven your breath. Kapalabhati is performed by taking short, sharp exhales through your nose and then allowing the inhalation to drop effortlessly back into the body. In this exercise, it's tempting to collapse the chest to assist the exhale; instead, keep the chest open and free and use the strength of the abdominals snapping in and up to create a strong, short exhalation.

Begin with a slow pace (about one breath per second). Go as slowly as feels comfortable, and build to a quicker pace over time.

- ▶ Sit comfortably on a cushion or chair with a tall, straight spine.
- ▶ Place your hands on your knees,
- ▶ Keeping your chest wide and open, inhale and exhale naturally and easily.
- ▶ After your next full exhale, inhale halfway.
- ▶ Using the abdominals to lift in and up, complete the exhale sharply out through the nose.
- ▶ Allow the inhale to drop in effortlessly.
- ▶ Repeat the assisted exhales through the nose at your own pace, allowing the inhale to drop in naturally each time. Keep your chest open and your throat and face soft.
- ▶ Repeat ten to fifteen times.
- ▶ When you have finished, take a few normal, slow breaths.
- ▶ Close your eyes and feel the increased warmth, energy, and vigor of your body.

BREATH PRACTICE
(Ujjayi):
FOR CALM STRENGTH

Ujjayi is practiced by finding a soft constriction through the back of the throat in order to make your breath slightly audible. Through Ujjayi, we can lengthen our breathing, make the inhale and exhale the same length, and smooth the texture of our breath.

- ▶ Sit comfortably on a cushion or chair with a tall, straight spine.

- ▶ Bring your palm in front of your mouth, and as you exhale, "fog" up your hand as if it were a mirror.

- ▶ Hear the audible smooth quality of this whispered "ahhhh" as you exhale.

- ▶ Continue to inhale through your nose, and exhale through your mouth on this whispered "ahhh" sound for several breaths until it feels natural.

- ▶ Place your hand back on your thigh.

- ▶ Now as you exhale, keep this soft constriction through your throat, but exhale through your nose rather than your mouth.

- ▶ Keep this soft constriction as you inhale through your nose. The inhale may take a bit more practice than the exhale at first.

- ▶ Continue to inhale and exhale smoothly with this internal whispered "ahhh." Make sure your jaw is relaxed.

- ▶ You can plug one or both ears, which will allow you to hear your breath more clearly.
- ▶ Close your eyes.
- ▶ Using Ujjayi, breathe smoothly, calmly, and slowly.
- ▶ If it is comfortable, lengthen the cadence of your breath by lengthening your exhale.
- ▶ If it is comfortable, you may begin to discover a natural pause between your inhale and your exhale.
- ▶ Enjoy the rhythmic sounds of your breath for several minutes.
- ▶ When you are ready, let go of the constriction in your throat and take a few natural, easy breaths.
- ▶ Bring your hands to your chest and take a moment to honor the calm strength of your body.

SUN BREATH

(Surya Bhedana):

FOR ENERGIZING

In yoga philosophy, the right nostril is connected to an energy channel that is activating and warming. In this breath technique, we stimulate this channel with our breath in order to awaken the activating energy in the body.

- ▶ Sit in a comfortable position on a cushion or on a chair.

- ▶ Bring the index and middle finger of your right hand to lightly touch the base of your thumb. By doing so, the thumb and ring finger now may form a pincer grip. This hand position is called *mrigi mudra*, or "deer seal," because it looks like a deer's antlers and is designed to help us seal and direct energy in our bodies.

- ▶ Place your thumb on the right side of the bridge of your nose, and your ring finger on the left side. You will find that by applying light pressure to each side, you can control the airflow into each nostril.

- ▶ Rest your left hand comfortably on your left thigh, with an option to join your thumb and index finger in a circle. This hand position is called *jnana mudra*, or "wisdom seal."

- ▶ Inhale and exhale through both nostrils.

- ▶ Block your left nostril and inhale slowly through your right.

- ▶ Exhale slowly through your left.

- ▶ Inhale slowly through your right.

- ▶ Exhale slowly through your left.

- ▶ Take about ten more rounds of this circular breath, inhaling through your right nostril and exhaling through your left.

- ▶ Release your nose, and allow your right hand to come down to your thigh, joining your thumb and forefinger together.

- ▶ Take several slow, easy breaths.

- ▶ When you're ready, press your hands together in front of your heart and sense any changes in the quality of your energy.

INSPIRATION & UPLIFTING

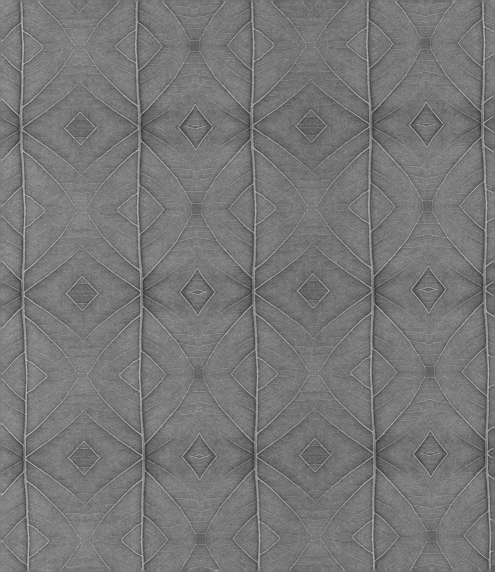

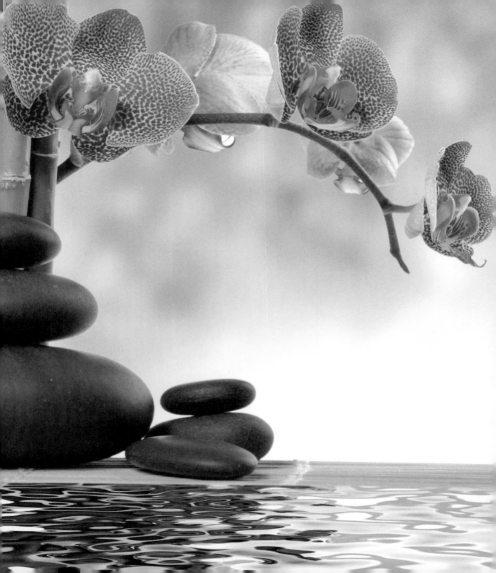

Remember your own magnificence.

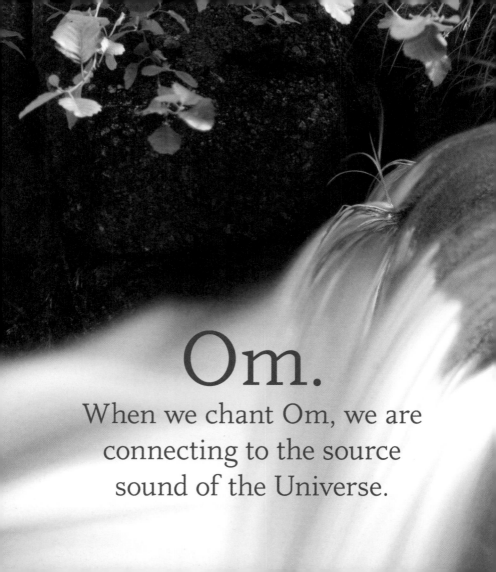

Om.

When we chant Om, we are connecting to the source sound of the Universe.

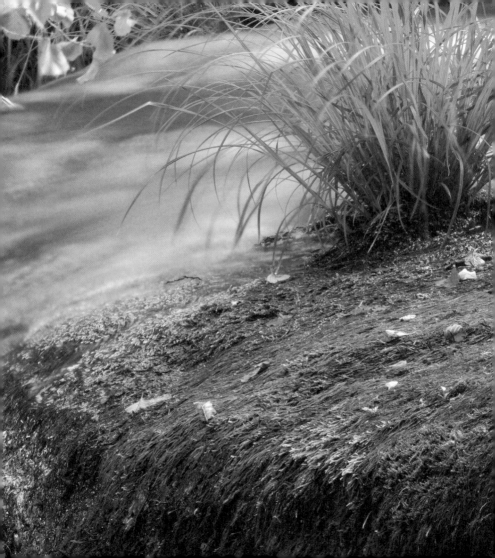

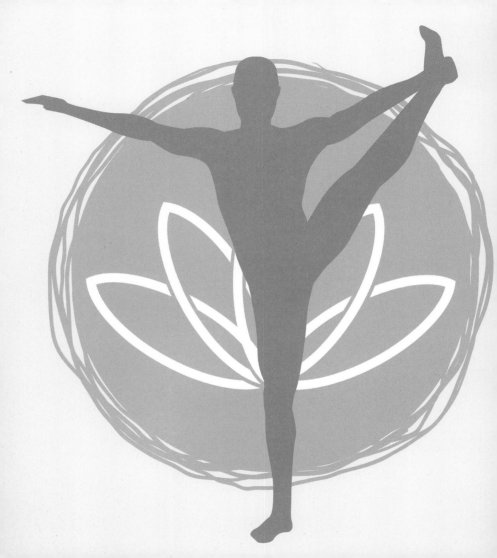

Did you know…

For most of its long history,
yoga has been a practice
of meditation. Only in the past
hundred years has yoga become
so focused on postures.

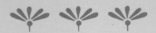

Tat Tvam Asi:
You are That.

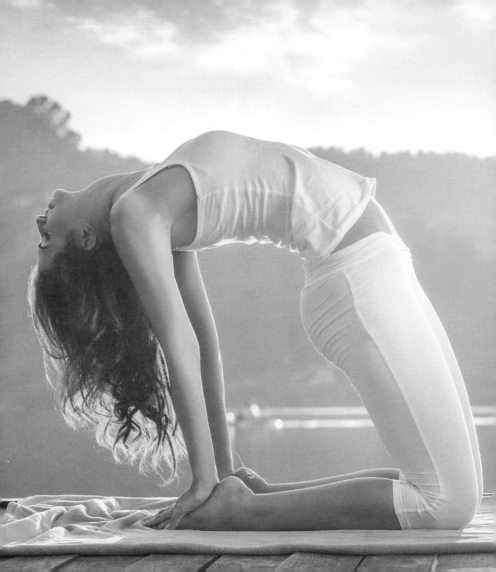

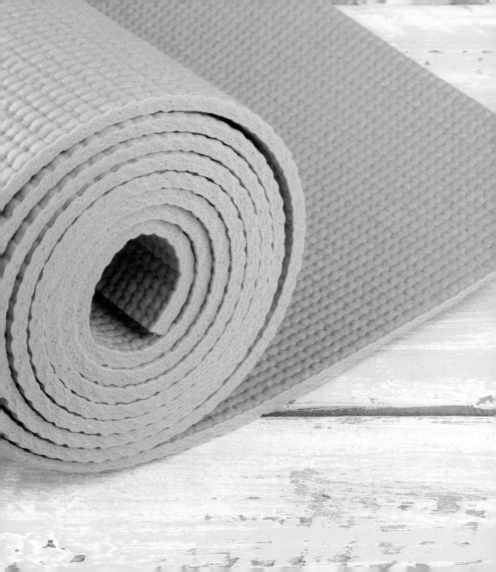

The yoga practice invites us
to return again and again
to the mat. Not for the sake
of self-improvement, but
to remove our confusion that
we are not already whole.

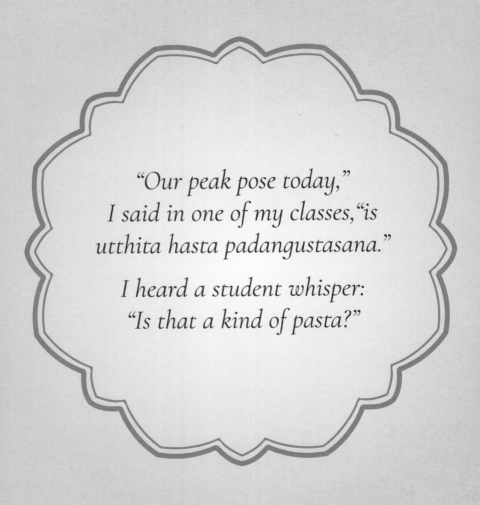

"Our peak pose today,"
I said in one of my classes, "is
utthita hasta padangustasana."

I heard a student whisper:
"Is that a kind of pasta?"

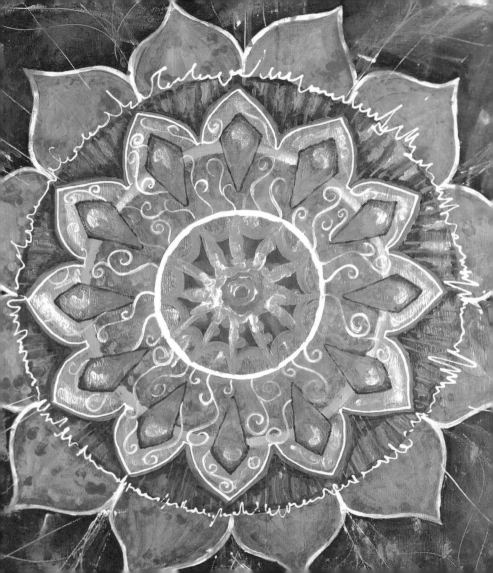

TRIANGLE POSE

(Trikonasana):

FOR OPENING

OPTIONAL PROPS: block or books

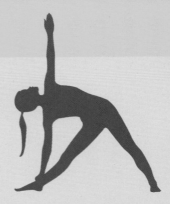

- ▶ Stand in the middle of your mat, facing the long side, and extend your arms. Step your feet wide so that your feet are beneath your wrists.

- ▶ From the top of your right thigh, turn your right thigh out so that your foot points directly to the top of your mat.

- ▶ Line up your front heel with the middle of your back arch and turn your back toes in slightly.

- ▶ Pull up strongly through both legs.

- ▶ Shift your hips towards your back heel and pull your right hip crease deeply into your body.

- ▶ Keeping both sides of your torso long, hinge from your hips and bring your right hand onto your shin (or onto a block or stack of books on the outside of your shin).

- ▶ Press firmly into your right big toe mound as you pull your right hip back and under you.

- ▶ Lengthen your tailbone and pull your front ribs to find evenness in the torso front and back.

- Take your left hand up to the sky in line with the shoulder.

- Depending on what is comfortable for your neck, look down, to the side, or up to your fingertips.

- Push your feet down into the floor and fully stretch your arms.

- Take three to five deep breaths.

- Look down, soften your front knee, and press through your feet to come up.

- Repeat on the second side.

SUN SALUTATION
(Surya Namaskar):

Sun salutations are a moving meditation, which uplift the body, mind, and spirit. Take each movement in your own time with your breath.

- Stand in Mountain Pose (*tadasana*) with your feet hip distance apart and parallel.

- As you inhale, reach your arms up to the sky (Upward Worship).

- As you exhale, forward fold and bring your fingers to the earth.

- As you inhale, bring your fingertips to your shins, and lift halfway up into a mini backbend.

- As you exhale, place your palms to the earth shoulder distance apart and step back into plank.

- Optional: Take a full breath in plank, and you have the option to lower your knees down for support.

- As you exhale, reach your heart forward, widen your collarbones, and slowly lower halfway (*chaturanga*) or fully down to the earth.

- As you inhale, reach your chest forward and up into Cobra or Upward Facing Dog.

- As you exhale, engage your core and reach your hips up and back to come into Downward Dog.

- Hug your hands and your forearms towards each other as you stretch your hips up and back to lengthen your spine.

- Take five deep breaths.

- At the end of your fifth exhale, step or walk your feet to the front of your mat.

- Inhale, bring your fingertips to your shins, and lift halfway up into a mini backbend.

- Exhale into a forward fold with your fingertips on the earth.

- Inhale, press through your feet, and reach your arms up into the sky (Upward Worship).

- Exhale your hands to your sides to come back into Mountain Pose.

- Repeat up to five times, and feel your whole body expand into this moving meditation.

UPWARD WORSHIP

(Utthita Hastasana):

FOR UPLIFTING YOUR POINT OF VIEW

Changing the state of our physical body can shift our mind and our feelings. In yoga terms, what we do with our physical body (*annamaya kosha*) has a ripple effect on our breathing (*pranaymaya kosha*) and our mind (*manomaya* and *vijnanamaya kosha*). Holding this simple pose has been shown to shift the chemistry of our hormones, reducing stress and increasing our confidence.

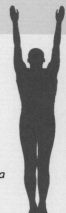

Change your body and change your mind.

▶ Stand in Mountain Pose (*tadasana*) with your feet hip distance apart.

▶ Lift your arms up into a wide V above your head and stretch through your fingertips.

▶ Root down strongly into the earth to stretch your arms further towards the sky, lengthening through the sides of your body.

▶ Relax the muscles at the base of your neck as you draw your upper arm bones back by your ears and open your chest expansively.

▶ Breathe into the open space of the front of your heart.

▶ Stay in this pose for two minutes, continuing to ground through your feet and stretch through the edges of your body.

▶ After two minutes, relax your arms and take few deep breaths.

Enjoy the transformation of your energy!

MEDITATION
(Ajna Chakra)
FOR CLARITY

▶ Find a comfortable seat with a tall spine on the floor, a cushion, or a chair.

▶ Allow your breathing to slow.

▶ Focus on the sensations of your breath until your body becomes calm.

▶ Visualize a white light softly glowing at your third eye. Your third eye is in your midbrain, located behind the spot just above and between your eyebrows. In yoga philosophy, Ajna, the Third-Eye Chakra, is the portal to self-realization and insight.

▶ If thoughts arise, come back to the vision of the white light.

▶ Remain in meditation for anywhere between five and twenty minutes.

▶ When you are finished, let go of the image from your mind.

▶ Take a few deep breaths.

▶ Rub your palms together to create some heat, then place your palms over your eye sockets and let the warmth of your hands move back into your skull.

▶ Bring your hands to your heart center and bow your head to your heart.

▶ Open your eyes, and take your time to come back into your body and your day.

MEDITATION
(Om)
FOR A HIGHER CONNECTION

▶ Find a comfortable seat with a tall spine on the floor, a cushion, or a chair.

▶ Allow your breathing to slow.

▶ Focus on the sensation of your breath until your body becomes calm and still.

▶ On your inhalation, feel the subtle opening and expansion of your body.

▶ On your exhalation, begin to imagine a slow internal chant of the sound *Om*.

▶ Inhale and feel open space.

▶ Exhale, and hear the internal sound of Om.

- ▶ Let the subtle vibration of the sound fill your body, nourishing your cells.

- ▶ Remain in meditation for five to twenty minutes.

- ▶ When you are finished, release the internal sound, and take a few deep breaths.

- ▶ Rub your palms together to create some heat, then place your palms over your eye sockets and let the warmth of your hands move back into your skull.

- ▶ Bring your hands to your heart center and bow your head to your heart.

- ▶ Open your eyes, and take your time to come back into your day.

MEDITATION

FOR INSPIRATION

- ▶ Find a comfortable seat with a tall spine on the floor, a cushion, or a chair.

- ▶ Allow your breathing to slow.

- ▶ Focus on the sensations of your breath until your body becomes calm.

- ▶ Bring to mind someone whom you admire greatly. This can be someone from history, the present, or someone who is close to you.

- As you visualize this person, bring to mind the qualities about them that inspire you.

- Allow the experience of this inspirational person to fill your consciousness.

- If your attention drifts, simply notice and come back to the person.

- Remain in meditation for five to twenty minutes.

- Take a moment to send a thank you to this person, and then release them from your mind.

- Take a few deep breaths.

- Bring your hands to your heart center and bow your head to your own heart.

- Open your eyes, and take your time to come back into your day.

We admire those individuals who reflect qualities that we already have. By meditating on someone who inspires us, we practice gratitude for that person, and also reaffirm those inspirational qualities in ourselves.

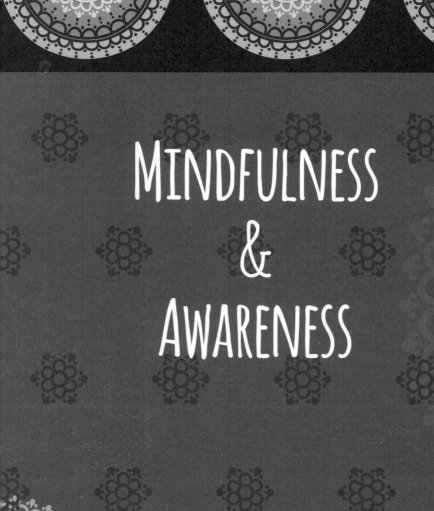

MINDFULNESS & AWARENESS

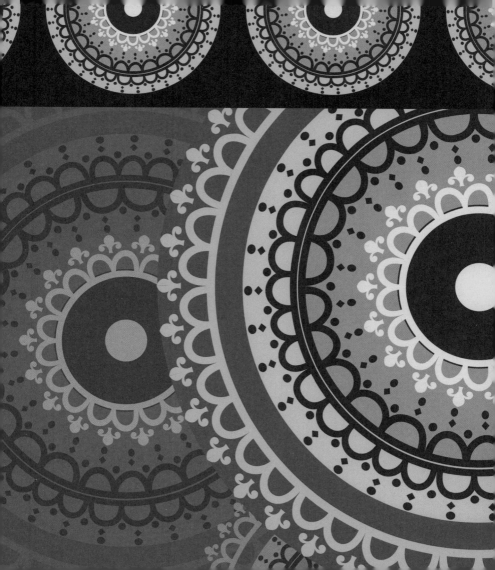

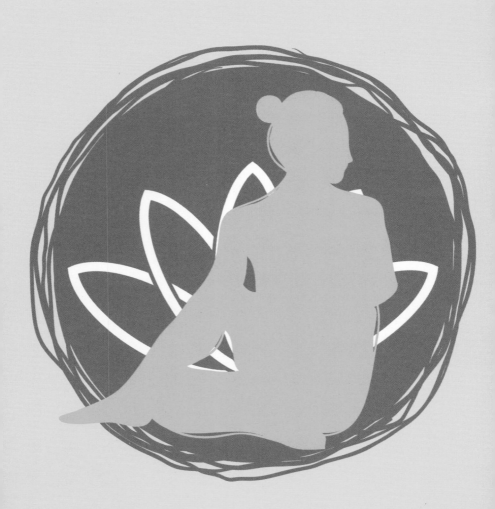

Did you know…

Yoga is traditionally
taught one on one?
Group classes are
a modern phenomena.

The world provides us with continual opportunities for practice. When we find ourselves in an emotional reaction, the Universe is giving us a wonderful opportunity to simply pause and feel. For a moment, practice letting go of the story and become aware of the sensations of your body. Can you rest in that space of just being?

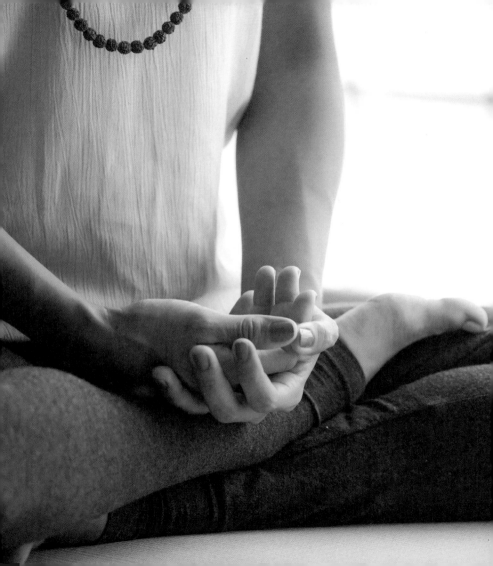

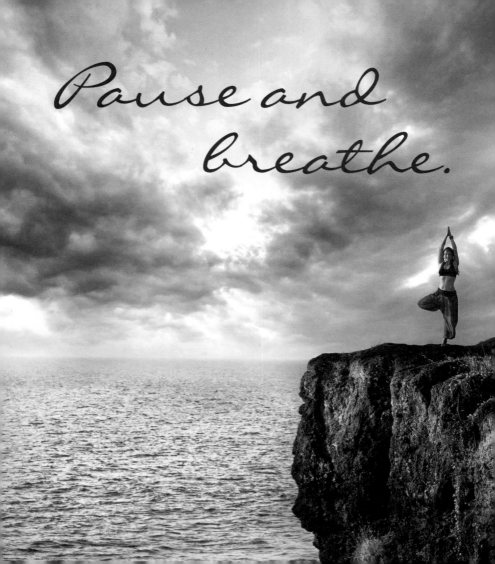

There is only now.

The Bhagavad Gita is a treasured Indian epic about a hero, Arjuna, who finds himself on the field of battle, about to go to war with his kinsmen over the throne. Although Arjuna's claim to the throne is just, he collapses in despair because he does not want to fight his own family. His charioteer reveals himself to be a god, Krishna, who counsels Arjuna to do his duty and fight. Krishna calls this kind of mindful action karma yoga, or "skill in action."

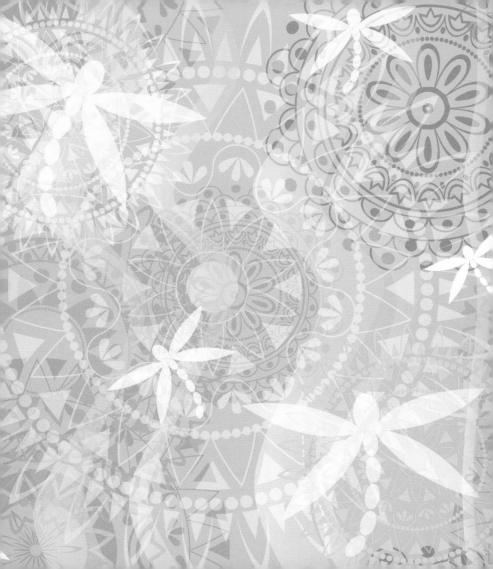

MINDFULNESS METER

The human mind loves to travel on autopilot. All too often, a day has gone by and we feel as if we were never quite in it! This simple mindfulness meter practice can helps us to catch ourselves throughout our day and "wake up" to the present moment.

▶ Set a timer to go off in hourly increments throughout your day. You can have the timer chime or buzz (depending on your surroundings).

▶ When the timer goes off, catch yourself! Were you awake or "asleep" to the present moment?

▶ Let the timer be a wake-up call to arrive again in the present moment.

By waking ourselves up every hour, we can become more aware of ourselves and mindful of our impact in our lives.

OPTIONS:

1. Keep a log of your hourly wake-up calls. How aware were you throughout the day?

2. Set the time for shorter intervals, such as fifteen or thirty minutes.

SAVOR YOUR FOOD

As you enjoy your meal, slow down to experience the texture, flavor, and spice of what you taste. Turn each mouthful into an opportunity to awaken your senses, and delight in the simple pleasures of the world.

EASY SEAT

(Sukhasana):

FOR MEDITATION

There are many ways to sit for meditation. Easy seat (*sukhasana*) is a very accessible and grounding position for many people. You may choose to sit on a yoga mat, blanket, or a clean floor.

OPTIONAL PROPS: block, pillow

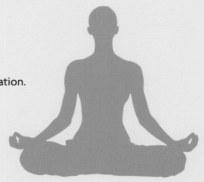

▶ Come into a cross-legged seat where you are crossing at your shins (rather than the ankles). Notice which shin you naturally cross in front. Switch your legs so that your "non-traditional" shin is in front. As you practice, make sure to alternate which leg is in front in order to create balance in the body.

▶ In this position, your ankles should be under your knees.

▶ The shins should be placed far enough away that when you look into your lap, there is an open, triangular space between your hips and legs.

▶ If your spine is rounding or the position is uncomfortable for any reason, sit on a block or a pillow to elevate your hips.

- Relax your legs fully. If your knees are high above your pelvis (even with a block), then come to sit on the edge of a chair.

- To find the best position for your pelvis, tilt your hips forward and backward. Make your rocks smaller and smaller until you find the center of the sitting bones. Sit on top of the sitting bones in the place that makes your spine feel the most supported and tall.

- Once you have found your seat, lift through the top of your head to lengthen your spine.

- Place your hands on your thighs and draw your upper arm bones back slightly to open your chest.

- Inhale and allow your collarbones to widen and your ribs to expand.

- As you exhale, feel the subtle lifting of the pelvic floor—the diamond shaped hammock of muscles that act as a sling between your sitting bones, tailbone, and pubic bone. Keep this very soft lifting of support. This is called the root lock (*mula bandha*), and it helps to harness the internal energy (*prana*) of your body, as well as keep you upright.

- Without diminishing the free and open space of your body, now see how relaxed your body can become. Soften your muscles, your face, your throat, and your eyes.

- Keeping the back of your neck long, gently tip your chin towards your chest until you feel a soft containment through the front of the throat, as if you were holding an orange beneath your chin. This is the chin lock (*jalandhara bandha*). It helps contain your body's internal energy (*prana*) and create a natural internal focus.

- Your body is now ready to meditate.

HERO'S POSE

(Virasana):

FOR MEDITATION

Hero's pose (*virasana*) can be practiced sitting
on blocks to give more space to the knees.

OPTIONAL PROPS: blocks or books

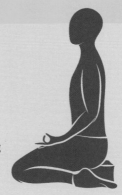

▶ Stack at least two blocks on top of each other.

▶ Come to sit on the blocks so that your ankles are hugging the outside
of the blocks and your thighs are parallel to each other.

▶ Ensure that your thighs are in line with your hips (rather than splaying
out). At this point, you can assess if you are sitting too high or too low.
Some of us may prefer more blocks and more space; others may
remove a block and sit on just one (or even between the heels with
their buttocks on the floor). As we want to be able to sit for at least
five minutes, choose a position that is comfortable for your body.

▶ If your ankles feel overstretched, you may place rolled up socks
between the front of your ankle and the floor.

▶ To find the best position for your pelvis, tilt your hips forward and
backward to feel your sitting bones against the blocks. Make your rocks
smaller and smaller to find the center of the sitting bones. You want

to sit on top of the sitting bones in the place that makes your spine feel the most supported and tall.

▶ Place your hands on your upper thighs. You can either place your palms up (to feel more receptive) or down (to feel more grounded).

▶ Draw your upper arm bones back to widen your collarbones.

▶ Inhale and feel your lungs and ribs expand.

▶ As you exhale, feel the subtle lifting of the pelvic floor – the diamond shaped hammock of muscles that act as a sling between your sitting bones, tailbone, and pubic bone. Keep this very soft lifting of support. This is called the root lock (*mula bandha*), and it helps to harness the internal energy (*prana*) of your body, as well as keep you upright.

▶ Without diminishing the free and open space of your body, now see how relaxed you can become. Soften your muscles, your face, your eyes.

▶ Keeping the back of your neck long, gently tip your chin towards your chest until you feel a soft containment through the front of the throat, as if you were holding an orange beneath your chin. This is the chin lock (*jalandhara bandha*). It helps contain your body's internal energy (*prana*) and create a natural internal focus.

▶ Your body is now ready to meditate.

THUNDERBOLT

(Vajrasana):

FOR MEDITATION

Thunderbolt (*vajrasana*) is a meditation pose where you sit on your shins.

OPTIONAL PROPS: pillow, bolster, or foam block

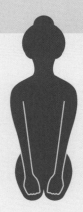

- ▶ Come onto all fours.
- ▶ Hug your ankles, shins, and knees together.
- ▶ Keeping your knees and feet together, exhale and sit back onto your heels. You may use your hands to pull the muscles of your calves down towards your ankles.
- ▶ If you find the position too compressing for your shins, you may place a pillow, bolster, or foam block between your shins and the floor.
- ▶ If your ankles feel overstretched, you may place rolled up socks between the front of your ankle and the floor.
- ▶ Sit on the center of your sitting bones so that your spine is lifting tall.
- ▶ Place your hands on your upper thighs by your hip creases to open your chest. You can either place your palms up (to feel more receptive) or down (to feel more grounded).
- ▶ Draw your upper arm bones back to widen your collarbones.

▶ Inhale and feel your lungs and ribs expand.

▶ As you exhale, feel the subtle lifting of the pelvic floor – the diamond shaped hammock of muscles that act as a sling between your sitting bones, tailbone, and pubic bone. Keep this very soft lifting of support. This is called the root lock (*mula bandha*), and it helps to harness the internal energy (*prana*) of your body, as well as keep you upright.

▶ Without diminishing the free and open space of your body, now see how relaxed you can become. Soften your muscles, your face, your eyes.

▶ Keeping the back of your neck long, gently tip your chin towards your chest until you feel a soft containment through the front of the throat, as if you were holding an orange beneath your chin. This is the chin lock (*jalandhara bandha*). It helps contain your body's internal energy (*prana*) and create a natural internal focus.

▶ Your body is now ready to meditate.

MEDITATION

FOR SOUND

▶ Find a comfortable seat with a tall spine.

▶ You may set a timer, or enjoy the meditation for as long as you wish.

▶ Close your eyes.

▶ Tune into the sound landscape of the world around you.

▶ Which sounds are near?

▶ Which sounds are far?

▶ Notice as the sounds you hear arise and dissipate.

▶ As each sound comes and goes, let go of your desire to label the sound and just hear the sound.

▶ Can you simply be with the open landscape of sound around you?

▶ As you complete your meditation, take a few deep breaths, and then slowly open your eyes to the world.

MEDITATION

FOR SIGHT

When we slow down to truly see what is around us, then the familiar transforms into unexpected opportunities for a fresh point of view.

▶ Take yourself on a neighborhood walk.

▶ As you travel down these familiar streets, slow down to see what is actually there.

▶ What are you seeing that you have never seen before?

▶ Open yourself to see the unexpected details of your landscape.

▶ Play with exploring color. Which colors do you see everywhere? Which shapes?

▶ When you come home, what looks different?

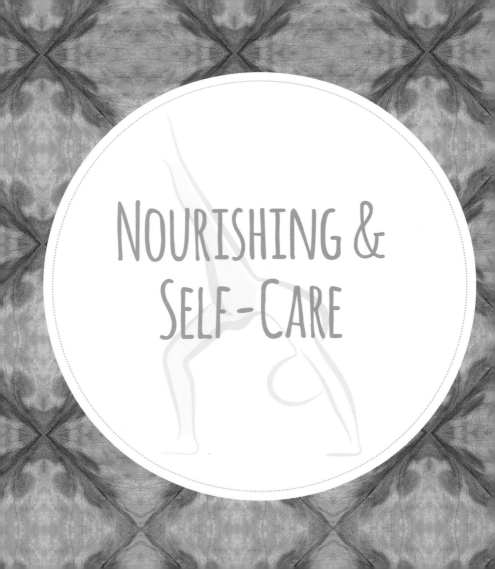

Nourishing & Self-Care

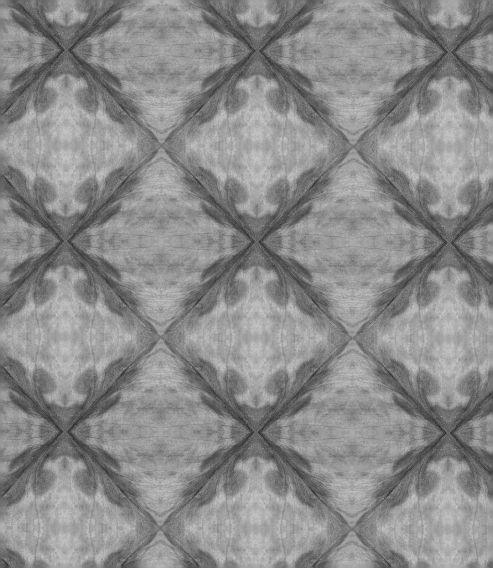

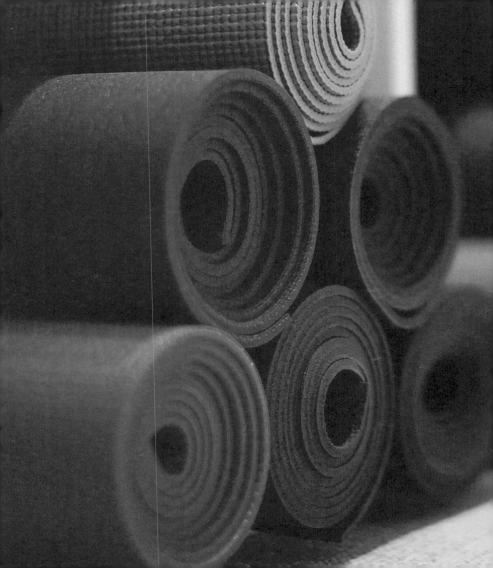

Dare to
increase your
capacity for
pleasure.

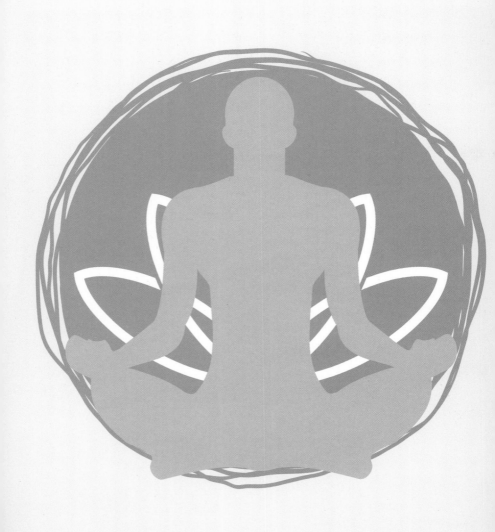

Did you know…

Some of the oldest yoga
texts are called Upanishads,
which means to "sit down near,"
reflecting the close relationship
of the teacher to the student.

Practicing self-care is like
washing the steps
of your own temple.

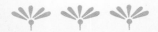

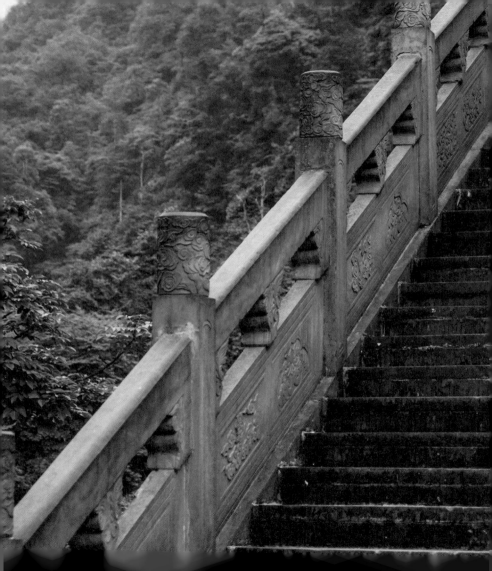

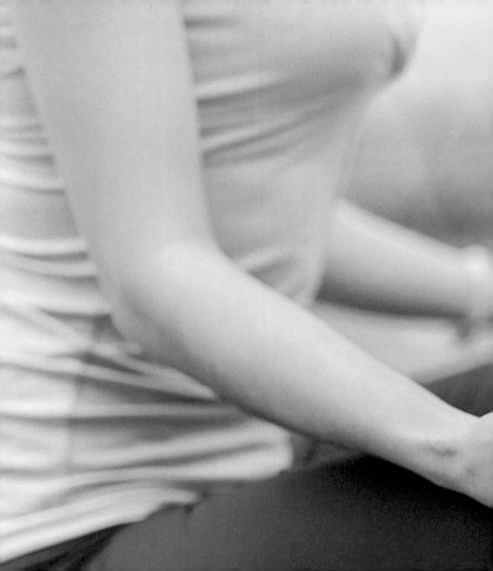

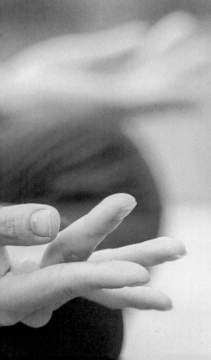

The mat is a space to nourish your unfiltered, authentic connection to yourself.

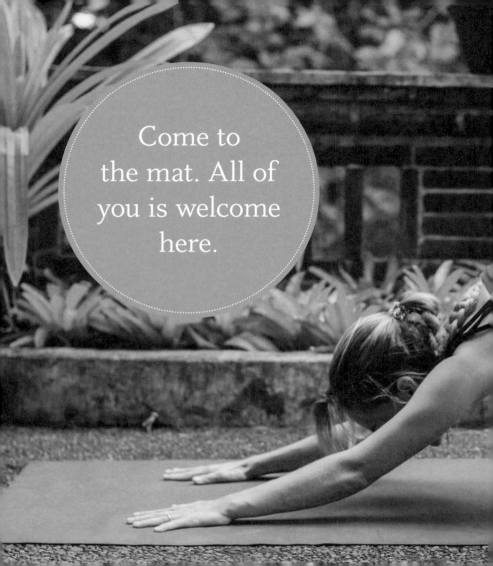

Come to the mat. All of you is welcome here.

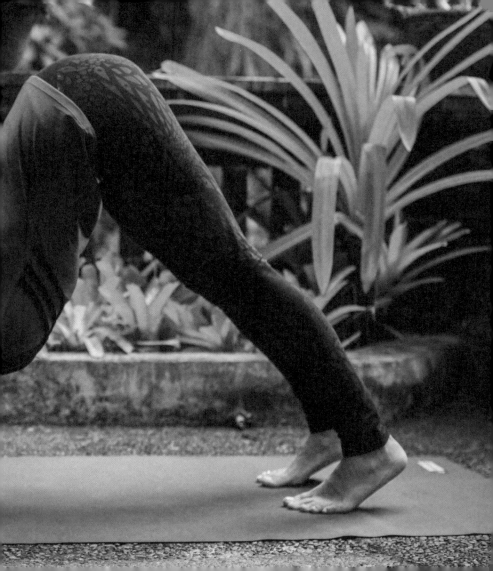

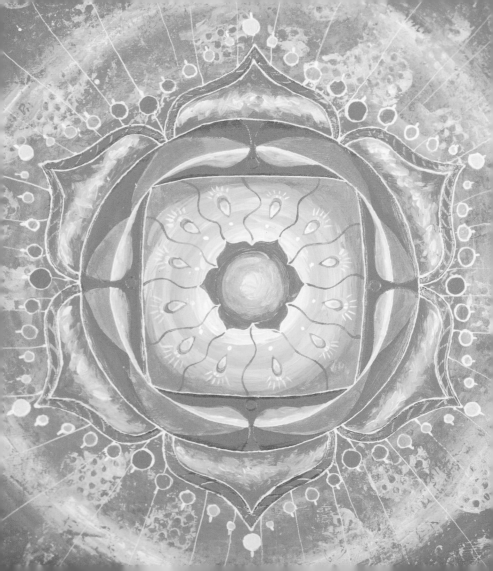

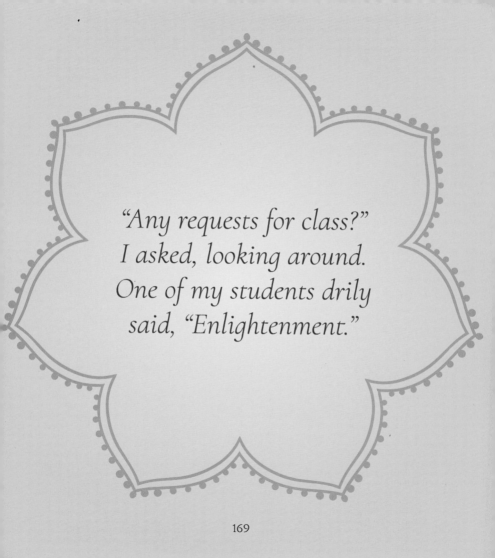

"Any requests for class?"
I asked, looking around.
One of my students drily
said, "Enlightenment."

Practice
radical
self-acceptance.

Be perfectly imperfect.

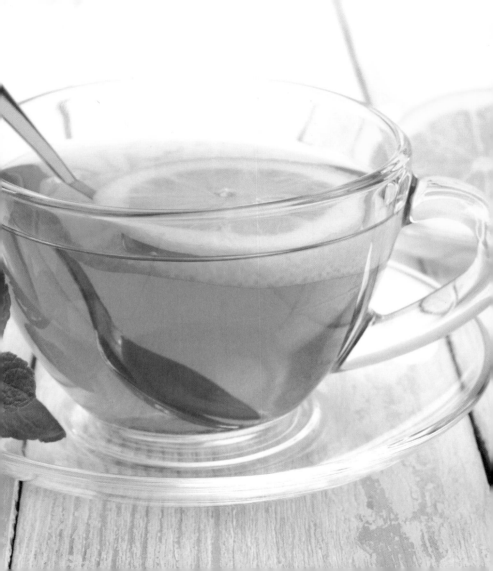

Take twenty minutes
just for you.

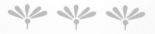

CAT/COW

(Marjaryasana/Bitilasana):

FOR NOURISHING THE SPINE

- ▶ Come onto your hands and knees.

- ▶ Place your palms under your shoulders and spread your fingers wide.

- ▶ Set your knees under your hips. You may curl your toes under or leave them flat.

- ▶ As you inhale, reach your heart forward through your arms, slide your shoulder blades down your back, and tip your sitting bones up to the sky.

- ▶ As you exhale, press through your hands, look towards your belly, and round the spine upwards.

- ▶ Continue this simple arching and rounding of your spine to find length through the front and back of your body.

- ▶ Link your breath with the movement, feeling your body open on the inhale, and contract on the exhale.

- ▶ Take five to ten cycles of cat and cow, then settle your hips back onto your heels and take Child's Pose.

OPTIONS:

DANCING CAT: Stretch a leg back on the inhale, and draw your knee into your chest as you exhale. Stay on the same side for several rounds before switching.

STRONG CAT: Stretch a leg back and also reach your opposite arms forward. As you exhale, challenge your balance by hugging your elbow and knee towards each other. Stay on the same side for several rounds before switching.

LOW LUNGE

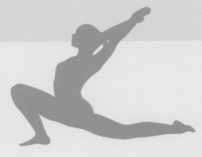

(Anjaneyasana):

THE ANTI-DESK POSE

Low lunge (*anjaneyasana*) is the perfect pose to relieve your body from the perpetual contraction of modern life (driving, deskwork, sitting).

▶ Come onto all fours with your hands just wider than your shoulders and your knees just behind your hips.

▶ Place your right foot by your right thumb.

▶ Bring your hands to your right thigh to lift your spine to vertical.

▶ Hug your thighs towards each other to square your hips.

▶ Lengthen your sitting bones down to floor and feel your core engage.

▶ Keep your tailbone heavy and begin to settle your hips forward and down to find a delicious stretch through the front of the left thigh.

▶ If your left knee moves in front of your left ankle, lengthen your stance so that your knee is stacked over your left heel.

▶ Draw your front ribs in, and reach your arms forward and up overhead in a wide "V".

▶ Press into your feet and hug your legs together to find stability.

▶ Draw your upper arms back and open the top corners of your chest into a mini backbend.

- ▶ Settle your hips earthward as you reach up through the length of your torso and stretch fully out through your fingertips.

- ▶ Enjoy three deep, opening breaths.

- ▶ As you exhale, bring your hands to your front thigh and then the earth. Step your right foot back and take a few breaths in Child's Pose before repeating on the other side.

LEGS UP THE WALL

(Viparita karani):

FOR TIRED LEGS

Legs up the Wall (*viparita karani*) is a pose that invites deep relaxation as it supports the nervous and circulatory systems. By inverting your legs' usual relationship to gravity, swelling through the ankles is eased and blood return to the heart is facilitated. This is a perfect pose for the end of day. Reclined poses are not recommended during the later stages of pregnancy.

OPTIONAL PROPS: strap, bolster, cushion, or block for under your head

- ▶ Sit about a foot away from the wall.

- ▶ Lie on your side and swing your legs up the wall.

- ▶ For tighter hamstrings, position your pelvis further from the wall (so legs are at a more inclined angle). If you have open hamstrings, position your pelvis closer to the wall. Take a position where your legs can comfortably relax, as this position is for relaxation rather than stretching.

▶ If your chin is tilting up, place a pillow or book under the back of your head so that your chin is level with the floor and the back of your neck is long.

▶ Allow your back body to completely relax into the floor, and let your legs relax and settle into the wall.

▶ Remain for about 5 minutes, letting yourself completely relax.

▶ To come out, bend your knees first into your chest, then slowly roll to one side. Take your time to come up, and sit quietly for a few moments.

NOTE: Depending on your body, your feet may become cool or may tingle as the blood moves from your extremities. Feel free to come out of the pose early, or bend and then straighten your legs to increase blood flow.

OPTIONS:

▶ To completely release any muscular tension through the hips, put a strap around your shins or your mid-thigh to hold your legs about hip distance apart. Then allow your legs to completely relax into its support.

▶ Placing a bolster under your hips is a nice option for creating a greater incline for your torso.

▶ If you find your chin is lifting to the sky, place a book or firm pillow under your head so that your chin is parallel to the floor.

PUPPY AT THE WALL

(Virabhadrasana III variation):

FOR SPINE LENGTHENING

Puppy at the Wall is my favorite yoga pose, perfect for lengthening and restoring the spine. This is an excellent pose for a momentary respite at home or in the office.

▶ Walk up to a wall, and place your hands shoulder distance apart at roughly the level of your hips.

▶ Step your feet back away from the wall until you bring your body into an L-shaped position with your feet directly under your hips.

▶ Look at your hands and make sure that your fingers are spread wide and pressing evenly into the wall.

▶ Still looking at your hands, press your palms into the wall and straighten your arms fully.

▶ Lower your head until it's just in line with your upper arms (not dropping).

▶ Bend your knees and strongly reach your hips back towards the center of the room.

▶ Find full spinal traction by pressing your hands forward as you reach your hips back.

- Keep your spine long by drawing your core in and up as you hug your shoulder blades towards each other.

- Keeping your spine long, press through your feet and slowly stretch your legs toward straight.

- Remain for another five to ten slow, deep breaths.

- Walk to the wall to stand up.

- Pause to feel the length and height of your body.

RECLINED BUTTERFLY

(Supta Baddha Konasana):

FOR LETTING GO

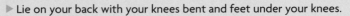

OPTIONAL PROPS: books or blocks for under the knees if needed, or a cushion or book for under your head. Reclined poses are not recommended during the later stages of pregnancy.

- Lie on your back with your knees bent and feet under your knees.

- Bring the soles of your feet together and allow your knees to open to the sides.

- If the stretch through the inner legs feels too strong, place blocks or books under your thighs to support the legs.

- Lift and reach your tailbone towards your heels to lengthen your lower back. If you feel any undue pressure through your lower back, then support your knees to be lifted higher or place a small cushion under your hips.

- If your chin is lifting towards the sky, then place a book or pillow under your head so that your chin is level with the floor and the back of your neck is long.

- Bring your hands to your belly or by your sides.

- Relax your face, your jaw, and your hips and allow your body to completely surrender to the floor.

- Remain in the pose for three to five minutes.

- When you're ready to come out, bring your hands to your outer thighs and use them to lift your legs ups.

- Slowly roll to your right side and take a few breaths.

- Look down and use your left hand to press yourself to a seated position.

- Take a few breaths and enjoy.

BREATH PRACTICE

FOR YOUR INNER SPACE

This simple combination of breath and movement helps us to reclaim the inner space of our body by releasing the tension that impedes the full expansion of our ribs.

▶ Come into Child's Pose and take a few breaths.

▶ As you exhale, feel your hips begin to settle and your lower back widen.

▶ Keeping your left hip firmly anchored, walk both hands towards the right side of your mat.

▶ Take several deep breaths into the stretch along the left side of your body to open the ribs.

▶ When you're ready, walk your hands back to center.

▶ Pause to take a breath and feel any difference now between your two sides.

▶ Keeping your right hip firmly anchored, now walk both hands towards the left side of your mat.

▶ Take several deep breaths into the stretch along the right side of your body to open the ribs.

▶ When you're ready, walk your hands back to center.

▶ Take a breath and feel the openness in the sides of your body.

- Walk your hands back to your knees and slowly rise to sit.
- Allow your shoulders to settle on your back.
- Take a few breaths and feel the new space that has opened through your ribs and lungs.

BREATH PRACTICE

FOR AWARENESS

- Find a comfortable seat so that your spine is tall.
- Close your eyes.
- Start with a few deep, nourishing breaths and generous exhalations.
- As you slowly inhale, feel the inner space of your body—belly, ribs, and chest—open and widen.
- As you exhale through your mouth, allow your body to relax, and release any stress from your day.
- As you continue to breathe, allow your breath to become quieter and calmer. It may become quite subtle.
- Lightly focus on the sensation of your breath, feeling your inner body expand on your inhale, and then soften on your exhale.
- If any thoughts arise, simply notice them and allow your attention to return to your breath.
- After a few minutes, gently open your eyes.

Stress Relief
&
Calming

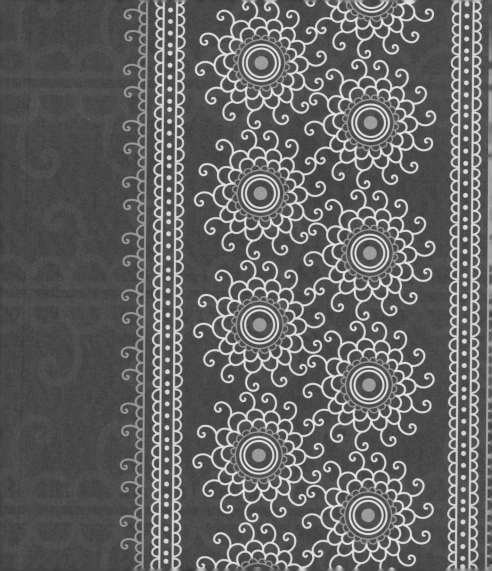

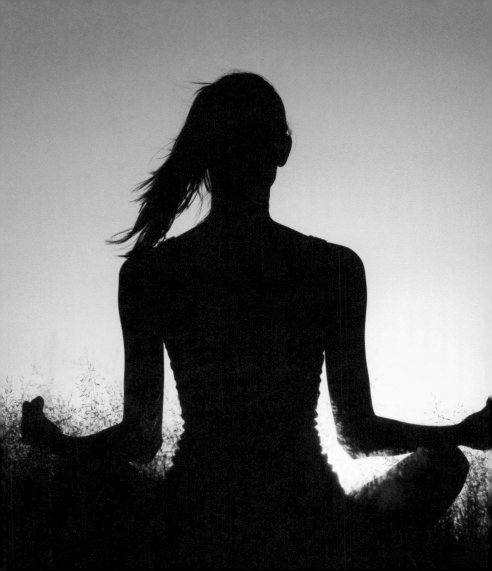

Take a deep breath.

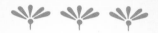

At any given moment,
you're only one
slow breath away from
a new point of view.

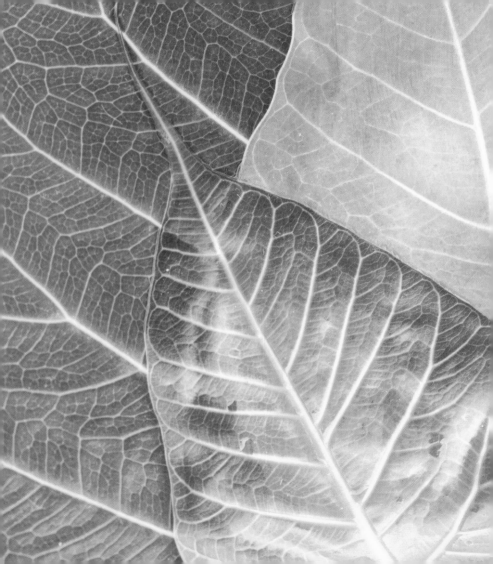

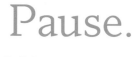

Pause.

Close your eyes.
Connect to your breath.
When you open your eyes,
what can you see that you
have never seen before?
What is fresh to your
point of view?

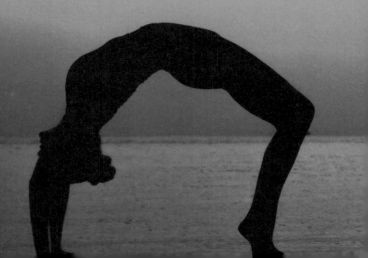

Much of our suffering stems
from the simple confusion
that we are our thoughts.
We become identified
with our racing minds.

When we pause, we can
recognize that there
is a great space within us.
We are the Presence
watching our thoughts.

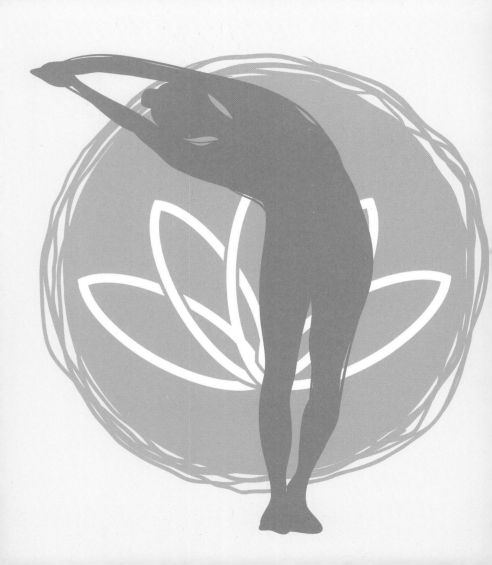

Did you know...

The irrigation of the nostrils
with salt water—now prescribed
by doctors for sinus issues—
was described as a yogic cleansing
technique over 500 years ago.

Take three
deep breaths.

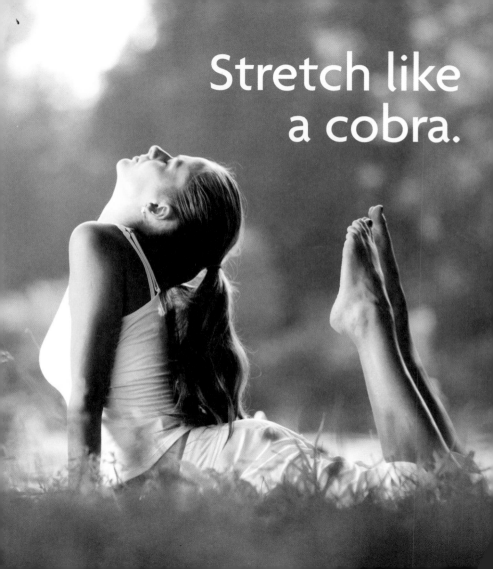

Stretch like
a cobra.

You are the home you seek.

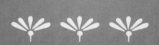

Slow down to feel.

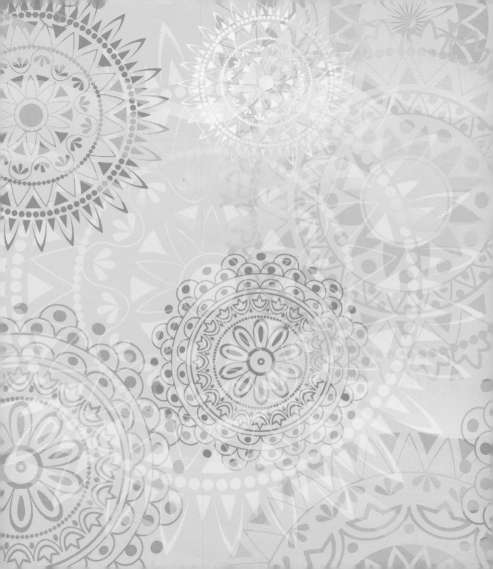

A new student came to practice at my teacher's studio, but didn't have a ride home. My yoga teacher offered to give her a lift. The student looked at her in surprise, "Why, that's so kind of you!" My yoga teacher paused. "Well, if yoga doesn't make you kinder, then what's the point?"

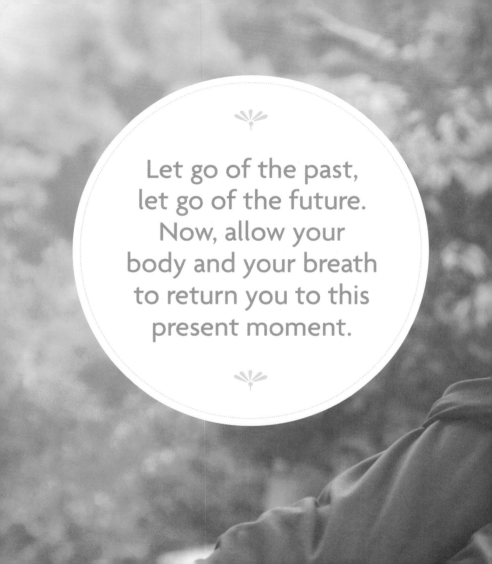

Let go of the past,
let go of the future.
Now, allow your
body and your breath
to return you to this
present moment.

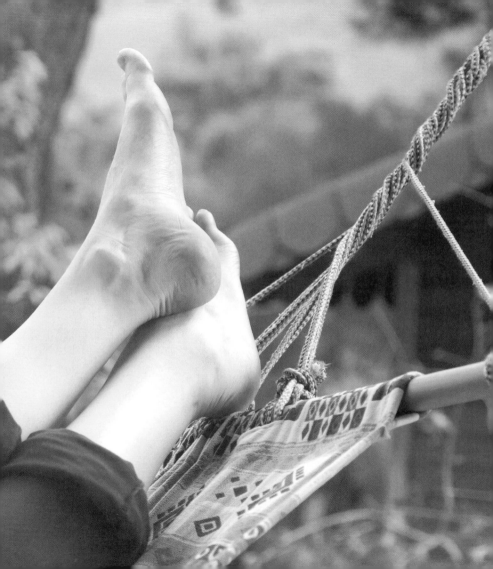

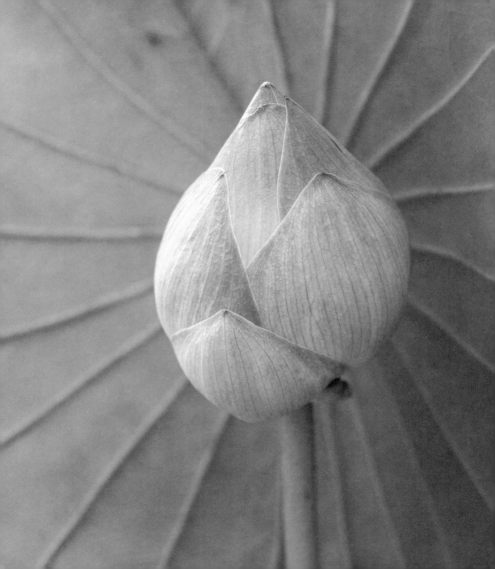

Shantih, shantih, shantih.
"Peace, peace, peace."

CHILD'S POSE

(Balasana):

FOR GROUNDING RELAXATION

Child's Pose (*balasana*) help us to ground the energy of our body, reconnect to our breath, and let go of the outside world. It is an ideal pose for settling anxiety and calming the nervous system.

▶ Sit with your toes together and your knees a little wider than hip-distance apart.

▶ Hinge forward from your hips to place your forehead on the earth. If the floor is too far away, then you can also place your forehead on a block or on your stacked hands.

▶ Allow your arms to fall where feels comfortable, either to the side of your head or back along the sides of your body.

▶ If your ankles are not used to stretching, you can roll up a washcloth or sock and place it between the tops of your ankles and the floor. If your knees aren't happy, then you can experiment with placing an evenly rolled thin towel behind the knee, lifting your body higher, or placing a cushion between your shins and hips.

▶ Check the position of your forehead against the floor and ensure that the skin of the forehead is wrinkling down towards the bridge of your nose rather than up.

- Relax all the muscles of your face, particularly the "expression muscles". Let your eyes, your jaw, your checks, and your lips soften.

- The center of your forehead is an important energy center for thinking and visualizing (*ajna chakra*). As you allow the head to get heavy, release thoughts and stresses from your head and into the earth.

- Your ribs should be supported by your thighs, but allow your belly to be soft and open.

- As you inhale, feel the breath move into your back ribs and lower back.

- As you exhale, allow any muscular tension to soften and let go.

- Remain in the pose for as long as feels nourishing.

- When you come out, take a few moments to stretch the backs of your knees by extending the legs back, or come into Downward Dog.

MOVING CHAIR
(Utkatasana):
FOR ACTIVE STRESS RELIEF

Sometimes we have a lot of energy in the body that needs to be released. This energy can manifest as anxiety, stress, fear, or anger. Moving Chair helps to dispel excess energy so that we can take care of our body's sympathetic nervous system and restore ourselves to a place of better balance.

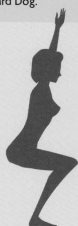

- Place your feet hip distance apart and parallel.

- Sit your hips back and down into Chair Pose and reach your arms forward and up.

- Take a big inhale.

- As you exhale loudly and vocally on "ha!", forward fold (keep your knees bent) and sweep your arms back behind you.

- Rebound and inhale slowly and fully as you come back into Chair, bringing your arms forward and up.

- Pause, then again, exhale loudly and vocally on "ha!", forward fold, and sweep your arms back behind you.

- Rebound back into Chair.

- Repeat this release technique up to five times, allowing yourself to dispel the excess energy of your body through your voice and movement.

- On your final rebound, settle into Chair for a couple slow breaths.

- Forward fold to release any tension through your shoulders or the back of your neck.

- Slowly roll up and breathe, feeling any energetic change through your body.

CORPSE POSE

(Savasana):

FOR LETTING GO

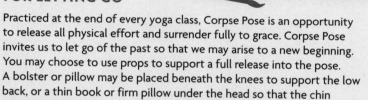

Practiced at the end of every yoga class, Corpse Pose is an opportunity to release all physical effort and surrender fully to grace. Corpse Pose invites us to let go of the past so that we may arise to a new beginning. You may choose to use props to support a full release into the pose. A bolster or pillow may be placed beneath the knees to support the low back, or a thin book or firm pillow under the head so that the chin is level to the floor. If you become cool easily, cover your body with a blanket. Lying flat on the back is not recommended for the later stages of pregnancy, but you can lay supported on your left side instead.

▶ Lie on your back with your legs extended long and hip distance apart.

▶ Turn your palms up and lay them down a few inches from your sides so that your chest is spacious and your collarbones are wide.

▶ Make any small adjustments that you may need (lengthening your tailbone, drawing your chin slightly down towards your chest) so that your body can fully relax into the floor.

▶ Close your eyes.

▶ Take several long, smooth breaths to fully release the tension from your body.

- ▶ Allow your front body to settle in your back body, and let yourself be completely supported by the earth.

- ▶ Soften your eyes, your face, your jaw, and your throat.

- ▶ Allow all thoughts to dissolve as you settle into your breath.

- ▶ Let your breath slow down and become soft and subtle. Your breath may eventually become almost imperceptible.

- ▶ Remain in this deeply nourishing pose for a least five minutes, or as long as you like.

- ▶ When you want to emerge from the pose, draw your knees into your chest and roll onto your right side. Cradle your head on your right arm and take a few breaths.

- ▶ When you're ready to sit, use your top hand to press yourself slowly to a comfortable seat.

- ▶ Take a few slow breaths.

- ▶ Bring your hands together in front of your heart, and bow your head to your hands to connect to your own inner wisdom.

- ▶ Slowly open your eyes and arrive freshly to this moment.

SEATED FORWARD FOLD

(Paschimottanasana):

FOR CALM

Forward folding soothes the nervous system.
If you are tight through your hamstrings and back,
sit on a cushion or pillow to elevate your hips.

OPTIONAL PROPS: cushion, strap

▶ Come to sit with your legs extended out in front of you, hip distance
apart. If you find that your low back is rounding and it is challenging
to sit upright, then you can either bend your knees or sit on a cushion
or block.

▶ Stretch your legs as fully as possible, and turn your toes upward
so that your feet are parallel.

▶ Press your thighs down to the earth.

▶ Place your fingertips on the mat beside your hips, roll your shoulders
back, and use the connection of your hands pressing down to lift
up through the sides of your waist.

▶ Keeping your chest broad, hinge forward from your hips.

▶ If you feel a strong stretch through the back line of your body,
then feel free to stay here.

- ▶ You may also place a strap around the balls of your feet to give you more support.

- ▶ If it is easy to keep your spine long and hinging forward, then bring your hands forward and hold onto your to your shins or feet.

- ▶ Keeping some light support through your core, hug your shoulder blades onto your back and gently reach your chest forward.

- ▶ As you inhale, lengthen your chest towards your toes.

- ▶ As you exhale, soften.

- ▶ Stay in the pose for about ten breaths.

- ▶ Inhale to lift your torso up.

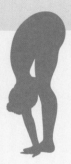

FORWARD FOLD

(Uttanasana):
FOR LETTING GO

- ▶ Stand with your feet hip distance apart and parallel.

- ▶ Press down through the four corners of both feet to lift your arches.

- ▶ Bring your hands to your hips.

- ▶ Inhale, roll your shoulders back, and lift your chest to lengthen your spine.

- As you exhale, bend your knees, and hinge forward from your hips.

- If possible, bring your chest onto your thighs so that your upper body is supported by your legs.

- When you have forward folded with a straight spine as deeply as you can, then allow your back to round, and release your head towards the floor.

- Hold onto opposite elbows, or place your hands on blocks to support your shoulders.

- Press through your feet, lift your sitting bones to the sky, and straighten your legs to your capacity.

- Take a few deep breaths, feeling the backs of your legs open and releasing any tension through your neck and jaw.

- Let your upper body hang heavy to lengthen your spine and release your back.

- After a few breaths, change the crossing of your elbows.

- Take three to five more deep breaths.

- To come out, soften your knees, bring your hands to your hips, and lift your shoulders.

- Press through your feet and slowly rise up to stand.

BREATH PRACTICE

FOR SELF-CONNECTION

Breath is life.

In Sanskrit, *prana* means both "air" and "life force." Our ability to control or expand our breathing has a direct effect on our energy and health. Through *pranayama* (breath-regulation techniques), we have a mainline to directly revitalizing and balancing our nervous systems.

There is actually no "right" way to breathe. Our body is a gloriously intelligent system that intuitively breathes to support us in a variety of circumstances, whether we are laughing, walking, sleeping, or running. However, over time and life, habitual tension and postural habits may begin to limit our body's natural options and freedom. By taking some time to unwind these patterns and reconnect to our breathing, we can restore and expand our body's innate capacity to find nourishment and energy in the midst of life's complexities.

OPTIONAL PROPS: blanket, foam block, book

This simple practice is designed to be done lying down.

▶ Lie on your back with your legs bent and your ankles under your heels. If it is comfortable for your body, take your feet as wide as your mat and allow your knees to drop in together. This will release your hips and widen your lower back. If your chin is lifting, then place a blanket, foam block, or small book underneath your head so that the back of your neck is comfortably long.

- ▶ Rest your hands on your belly.

- ▶ Relax your face, your eyes, and your jaw.

- ▶ Take a few natural breaths and expansive exhales.

- ▶ Allow your chest to remain still, and begin to breathe into the soft space of your belly.

- ▶ Stay relaxed and allow your breath to be as full or as shallow as feels natural.

- ▶ Continue to feel the breath move under your hands as you inhale and exhale. Notice how this feels.

- ▶ After a minute or so, let go and take a natural breath.

- ▶ Now, keeping your belly still, begin to invite the breath to move through your chest and your ribs. You may find it helpful to place your hands on your ribs or chest.

- ▶ Feel your breath move through the front, sides, and backs of your ribs. You may even feel the breath up into your collarbones.

- ▶ Notice how this feels. Notice any difference in the sensations of the two different breathing styles (one breathing pattern may feel very habitual, or very unfamiliar).

- ▶ After a minute or so, let go of your chest breathing and take a few natural breaths.

- ▶ Sense any change that you feel in your body.

- ▶ To come out, roll over onto your left side and pause, cradling your head in your left arm.

▶ Look down and keep your body relaxed as you use your right hand to press up to sit.

▶ Take a few breaths in a seated position to transition back to your day.

BREATH PRACTICE

FOR EXPANSION

Full, complete breath.

Building on your Breathing Practice for self-connection, this full, complete breath combines belly and the chest breathing to increase your internal space and calm the nervous system. It can be done immediately after the Breathing Practice for self-connection.

OPTIONAL PROPS: blanket, foam block, book

▶ Lie on your back with your legs bent and your ankles under your heels. If it is comfortable for your body, take your feet as wide as your mat and allow your knees to drop in together. This will release your hips and widen your lower back. If your chin is lifting, then place a blanket, a foam block, or a small book underneath your head so that the back of your neck is comfortably long.

▶ Rest your hands on your belly.

▶ Relax your face, your eyes, and your jaw.

▶ Take a few natural breaths and expansive exhales.

214

- ▶ Inhale, and then exhale completely.
- ▶ Breathe into your belly, and then continue to fill up and breathe through your ribs, chest, and upper chest.
- ▶ Pause.
- ▶ Exhale slowly and completely.
- ▶ Inhale again, beginning with a belly breath and then continuing to inhale into the lower ribs, side ribs, and upper chest.
- ▶ Pause.
- ▶ Exhale slowly and completely.
- ▶ Repeat five to ten more times.
- ▶ Let go of controlling your breath, and take a few natural inhales and exhales.
- ▶ Feel any change in your body.
- ▶ To come out, roll over onto your left side and pause, cradling your head in your left arm.
- ▶ Look down and keep your body relaxed as you use your right hand to press up to sit.
- ▶ Take a few breaths in a seated position to transition back to your day.

BREATH PRACTICE

FOR FINDING SPACE

This gentle, three-part breath practice (*viloma*) is a beautiful way to find more space for ourselves, both physically and mentally. If you find yourself in a stressful moment during your day, this breathing technique can immediately calm the body and mind, and help change your point of view. And the lovely thing is that no one needs to know that you're doing it.

▶ Find a comfortable seat with a tall spine.

▶ Close your eyes.

▶ Take a few moments and make a transition from thinking to feeling.

▶ Take a few natural, easy breaths.

▶ Exhale fully.

▶ Inhale into the space of your belly. Pause.

▶ Inhale into the space of your low ribs. Pause.

▶ Inhale into your upper chest and upper back. Pause.

▶ Exhale out slowly. This is one round.

▶ Repeat this interrupted breath cycle another five to ten times.

▶ Release the breath control and allow your body to breathe naturally.

▶ Sense any changes in your energy or breath sensation.

▶ When you are ready, slowly open your eyes.

MOON BREATH

(Chandra Bhedana):

FOR CALMING

In yoga philosophy, the left nostril is associated with an energy channel that is cooling and calming. In this breath technique, we stimulate the left channel with our breath in order to awaken this nourishing and calming energy in the body.

▶ Sit in a comfortable position on a cushion or chair.

▶ Bring the index and middle finger of your right hand to lightly touch the base of your thumb. By doing so, the thumb and ring finger now form a pincer grip. This hands position is called *mrigi mudra*, or "deer seal," because it looks like a deer's antlers and is designed to help us seal and direct energy in our bodies.

▶ Place your thumb on the right side of the bridge of your nose, and your ring finger on the left side. You will find that by applying light pressure to each side, you can control the airflow into each nostril.

▶ Rest your left hand comfortably on your left thigh, with an option to join your thumb and index finger in a circle. This hand position is called *jnana mudra*, or "wisdom seal".

▶ Inhale and exhale through both nostrils.

▶ Block your right nostril and inhale slowly through your left.

▶ Exhale slowly through your right.

▶ Inhale slowly through your left.

▶ Exhale slowly through your right.

▶ Take about ten more rounds of circular breath, inhaling through your left and exhaling through your right.

▶ Release your nose, and allow your right hand to come down to your thigh, joining your thumb and forefinger together.

▶ Take several slow, easy breaths.

▶ When you're ready, press your hands together in front of your heart and enjoy any changes in the quality of your energy.

INDEX

ABOUT THE AUTHOR

Rachel is the Director of Teachers' College and Development at YYoga, Canada's largest yoga company headquartered in Vancouver, BC. Raw and wry, she loves bringing yoga philosophy to life by blending candid storytelling with a mischievous sense of humor. She is passionate about helping people pursue their passion and potential. In addition to writing a 200 and 300 hour yoga training, she has logged thousands of hours as a mentor and teacher trainer. A total nerd, she earned her Masters of Fine Arts in Acting, her Masters of Science in Instructional Design, and her BA from Columbia University.

Rachel loves writing and contributes regularly to Yoga International and the Huffington Post. She shares her knowledge exuberantly; come meet her and enjoy her tips, classes, and musings at www.rachelyoga.com.

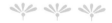

About Cider Mill Press Book Publishers

Good ideas ripen with time. From seed to harvest, Cider Mill Press brings fine reading, information, and entertainment together between the covers of its creatively crafted books. Our Cider Mill bears fruit twice a year, publishing a new crop of titles each spring and fall.

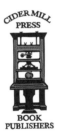

"Where Good Books Are Ready for Press"

Visit us on the Web at
www.cidermillpress.com
or write to us at
PO Box 454
12 Spring St.
Kennebunkport, Maine 04046